OPTICAL FORMULAS
TUTORIAL

Optical Formulas Tutorial

Ellen D. Stoner, M.A.L.S., ABOM
Opticianry Program Director,
Durham Technical Community College,
Durham, North Carolina

Patricia Perkins, B.S.c. (Hons), FBCO
Former Opticianry Program Director,
Durham Technical Community College,
Durham, North Carolina

BUTTERWORTH–HEINEMANN

Boston • Oxford • Johannesburg • Melbourne • New Delhi • Singapore

Butterworth–Heinemann supports the efforts of American Forests and the Global ReLeaf program in its campaign for the betterment of trees, forests, and our environment.

Library of Congress Cataloging-in-Publication Data

Stoner, Ellen D., 1947–
    Optical formulas tutorial / Ellen D. Stoner, Patricia Perkins.
      p.   cm.
    Includes bibliographical references and index.
    ISBN 0–7506–9913–2 (alk. Paper)
    1. Ophthalmic lenses. 2. Mathematics—Formulas. 3. Optics.
  4. Physiological optics. I. Perkins, Patricia, 1947– .
  II. Title.
  RE961.S97 1997
  617.7′52—dc21

                                           97–14338
                                              CIP

British Library Cataloguing-in-Publication Data
A catalogue record for this book is available from the British Library.

The publisher offers special discounts on bulk orders of this book.
For information, please contact:
Manager of Special Sales
Butterworth–Heinemann
313 Washington Street
Newton, MA 02158–1626
Tel: 617-928-2500
Fax: 617-928-2620

For information on all Butterworth–Heinemann medical publications available, contact our World Wide Web home page at: http://www.bh.com/med

10 9 8 7 6 5

Printed in the United States of America

CONTENTS

PREFACE

This text was originally designed to accompany an intensive seminar style review of formulas and basic ophthalmic optics information. Applicants for the North Carolina State Boards for Opticianry Licensure were the original target audience. The original project was conceived and written by Patricia Perkins, former Program Director of the Opticianry Department at Durham Technical Community College. The initial reaction from the intended audience was extremely positive.

As the text grew, the need for a comprehensive basic description of formulas without the many pages of discussion necessary for a comprehensive textbook became apparent. Thus, this text has grown to encompass most of the formulas that underlie basic ophthalmic optics theory. This text is intended to be a *formula reference*, not a stand-alone text.

Because the original intention was to help licensure applicants in an examination such as the ABO Masters exam which allows calculators but not charts, this text does not cover the non-formula techniques that are used in the field. An example would be prism resolving charts and graphs. For this reason, there are many techniques which are highly recommended to the practicing optician that are not a part of this tutorial.

This book starts with a review of basic math. The whole book is intended as a review, not a stand-alone text; this statement is particularly true of the math section. If *any* of the first section is unfamiliar or downright foreign, please discuss taking a math course with a counselor at your friendly local community college! Section I is intended for those readers who have basic math skills and just need a brush-up on the arithmetic. For a concentrated brush-up on math skills, see the Durham Technical Community College basic course OPH101 *Math for Opticians* on the Internet at **http://open.dtcc.cc.nc.us/opticianry/oph101**

If you are familiar with optical theory turn directly to any subject of interest in this book. If you are unfamiliar with the theory, or need an overall review, we recommend reading the text and performing the exercises in the order given.

Most of the subjects covered in Sections II through IV are covered in more detail in the Durham Technical Community College Opticianry course OPH141 *Optical Theory 1*, which is available on the Internet. The address for the assignment page of this 3 semester credit course is **http://open.dtcc.cc.nc.us/opticianry/oph141/**

Because we are used to specifying dioptric powers in quarter or eighth diopter steps, some opticians automatically round every dioptric value to the closest eighth. This rounding is valid for any power that we are going to make, order, verify, dispense, or record in the wearer's file. In many of the exercises and examples in this book we will round to hundredths, not to eighths. Rounding to hundredths occurs when the result of the calculation is an effective or actual power that will *not* be made, ordered, dispensed, or recorded in the wearer's file. Frequently we will be using the result for another formula or calculation, such as using the result of the oblique meridian formula in Prentice's rule for computing a prism amount. Other values, such as degrees, millimeters of thickness, and prism powers, will be rounded to the significance that we believe is supported by the accuracy of our customary equipment. We will indicate in each section the significance to which we are rounding. You are welcome, when using the formulas, to round to the significance that you consider valid.

We would like to thank the licensure applicants who attended the review seminars and the students in the degree program for their feedback. In particular, we would like to thank Margaret Rosar, Steven Gregory, and Nancy Sherrill, who have spent a great deal of time finding typing and calculating errors.

We enjoy receiving feedback on this text, and we would like to hear from you.

Ellen Stoner
Patricia Perkins

SECTION I: MATH REVIEW

Please work the exercises in this section completely. If any part of this math is new to you, or if you do not understand where the answers came from, please seek help with the basic algebra and math before you attempt to understand the use of our formulas. Some libraries have math tutors available. Most Community Colleges have people and courses who can help you improve your basic math and algebraic skills.

REVIEW OF ADDITION OF SIGNED NUMBERS

1. When adding numbers with the same signs, add the amounts and give the result their common sign.

EXAMPLE:

$$(-3.00) + (-2.00) = -5.00:$$ Since both numbers are negative, add 3 and 2, and use their common negative sign.

2. When adding numbers with different signs, subtract the amounts and give the result the sign of the larger number.

EXAMPLE:

$$(-3.00) + (+2.00) = -1.00:$$ Since they have different signs, subtract 2 from 3, leaving 1, and give the result a negative sign because the larger number, 3, is negative.

EXERCISES:

1. $(+1.00) + (+1.00) =$ _____

2. $(-1.00) + (-1.00) =$ _____

3. $(+3.00) + (+1.50) =$ _____

4. $(+3.00) + (-1.50) =$ _____

5. $(-4.50) + (-2.00) =$ _____

6. $(-4.50) + (+2.00) =$ _____

7. $(+7.50) + (-6.00) =$ _____

8. $(-3.25) + (+8.12) =$ _____

9. $(-10.00) + (-4.50) =$ _____

10. $(+6.75) + (+1.25) =$ _____

REVIEW OF SUBTRACTION OF SIGNED NUMBERS

To subtract signed numbers, change the sign of the subtracted number and add it.

EXAMPLE:

$$(+2.00) - (-4.00) = (+2.00) + (+4.00) = +6.00$$
$$(-3.00) - (-2.00) = (-3.00) + (+2.00) = -1.00$$
$$(-3.00) - (+2.00) = (-3.00) + (-2.00) = -5.00$$

EXERCISES:

1. $(+1.00) - (+1.00) = $ _____

2. $(-1.00) - (-1.00) = $ _____

3. $(+3.00) - (+1.50) = $ _____

4. $(+3.00) - (-1.50) = $ _____

5. $(-4.50) - (-2.00) = $ _____

6. $(-4.50) - (+2.00) = $ _____

7. $(+7.50) - (-6.00) = $ _____

8. $(-3.25) - (+8.12) = $ _____

9. $(-10.00) - (-4.50) = $ _____

10. $(+6.75) - (+1.25) = $ _____

REVIEW OF MULTIPLICATION OF SIGNED NUMBERS

1. When multiplying numbers with the same signs, the result is positive.

EXAMPLE:

$(-3.00)(-2.00) = +6.00$, because 3×2 is 6, and the numbers have the same signs.

2. When multiplying numbers with different signs, the result is negative.

EXAMPLE:

$(+3.00)(-2.00) = -6.00$, because 3×2 is 6, and the numbers have different signs.

EXERCISES:

1. $(+1.00)(+1.00) = $ _____

2. $(-1.00)(-1.00) = $ _____

3. $(+3.00)(+1.50) = $ _____

Optical Formulas Tutorial

4. $(+3.00)(-1.50) =$ _____

5. $(-4.50)(-2.00) =$ _____

6. $(-4.50)(+2.00) =$ _____

7. $(+7.50)(-6.00) =$ _____

8. $(-3.25)(+8.12) =$ _____

9. $(-10.00)(-4.50) =$ _____

10. $(+6.75)(+1.25) =$ _____

REVIEW OF DIVISION OF SIGNED NUMBERS

1. When dividing numbers with the same signs, the result is positive.
EXAMPLE:

$(-3.00)/(-2.00) = +1.50$, because 3/2 is 1.5, and the numbers have the same signs.

2. When dividing numbers with different signs, the result is negative.
EXAMPLE:

$(-3.00)/(+2.00) = -1.50$, because 3/2 is 1.5, and the numbers have different signs.

EXERCISES: (Round to two decimal places.)

1. $(+1.00)/(+1.00) =$ _____

2. $(-1.00)/(-1.00) =$ _____

3. $(+3.00)/(+1.50) =$ _____

4. $(+3.00)/(-1.50) =$ _____

5. $(-4.50)/(-2.00) =$ _____

6. $(-4.50)/(+2.00) =$ _____

7. $(+7.50)/(-6.00) =$ _____

8. $(-3.25)/(+8.12) =$ _____

9. $(-10.00)/(-4.50) =$ _____

10. $(+6.75)/(+1.25) =$ _____

ROUNDING

Most answers will need to be rounded to a particular significance. Do not round intermediate results; wait until you have a final answer to round. Look at the NEXT digit to the right of the digit you are rounding to. If it is a 4 or less, drop it and all digits to the right of it. If it is a 5 or more, increase the digit to the left by one, and drop all other digits to the right.

EXAMPLES:

Round to mm: 12.345mm → 12mm (The answer will be either 12 or 13. The next digit to the right is 3, which is '4 or less', so the .345 is dropped.)

Round to one-hundredths: +12.5862 → +12.59 (The one-hundredth place is an 8. The next digit to the right is 6, which is '5 or more'; add 1 to the 8 and drop the 62.)

Round to tenths: 6.74999 → 6.7 (The 7 is in the tenths place. The next digit to the right is 4, which is '4 or less', so the 4999 is dropped.)

ROUNDING DIOPTERS

When ordering or recording diopters, we use one-eighth diopter steps. Look for the dioptric step that the answer is the closest to. The dioptric steps are 0.12, 0.25, 0.37, 0.50, 0.62, 0.75, 0.87, 0.00. (See page 31.)

EXAMPLES:

Change to eighths: 0.15 → 0.12. (0.15 is 0.03 from 0.12, and 0.10 from 0.25. Therefore it will be changed to 0.12.)

Change to eighths: +8.326745 → +8.37 (.326745 is closer to .37 than it is to .25.)

EXERCISES:

Round to two decimal places:

    1. 132.5743   _____

    2. 0.455555   _____

    3. 1.56   _____

Round to whole numbers:

    4. 5.500   _____

    5. 4.499999   _____

    6. 8.9   _____

Change to eighths:

    7. −6.654   _____

    8. +0.24106   _____

    9. −3.30   _____

METRIC CONVERSIONS

A meter may be divided into parts. It is divided into tenths, hundredths, thousandths, etc.

METER ↔ DECIMETER ↔ CENTIMETER ↔ MILLIMETER

> m → dm → cm → mm
> 1.m = 10.dm = 100.cm = 1000.mm
> When converting from meters to centimeters or millimeters,
> move the decimal point to the right.
>
> m ← dm ← cm ← mm
> .001m = .01dm = .1cm = 1.mm
> When converting from millimeters or centimeters to meters,
> move the decimal point to the left.

EXAMPLES:

$\qquad$ 5.35m = 535cm = 5350mm

$\qquad$ 267mm = 26.7cm = 0.267m

EXERCISES: (Do not round.) .

1. Convert 5m to mm. $\qquad$

2. Convert 2m to cm. $\qquad$

3. Convert 50cm to mm. $\qquad$

4. Convert 2mm to cm. $\qquad$

5. Convert 2.45mm to m. $\qquad$

6. Convert 4.5cm to mm. $\qquad$

7. Convert 4.5cm to m. $\qquad$

8. Convert 80.5mm to m. $\qquad$

ENGLISH-METRIC CONVERSIONS

A yardstick is 3 feet or 36 inches long. A meter stick would be just slightly longer than a yardstick: it is 39.37 inches long. Therefore, 1m = 39.37in. Many times, it is more convenient to remember the approximation 1m ≈ 40in. If you have a ruler with both inches and mm on it, you will notice that one inch is just over 2.5cm long. In fact, 1in = 2.54cm = 0.0254m.

EXAMPLES: What would a 5 1/2 inch temple measure on a mm ruler? We have seen that 1in = 2.54cm = 25.4mm. Multiply both sides of the equals sign by 5.5:

$\qquad$ (5.5) (1in) = (5.5) (25.4mm) = 139.7mm = 140mm.

How many inches are there in 1/2 meter?

$1m \approx 40in$. Multiply both sides of the equals sign by 0.5:

$(0.5)(1m) = (0.5)(40in) = 20in$.

If the answer is asked for in feet, convert to inches and divide the answer by 12. If the problem is in feet, multiply by 12 to get inches, then convert. Most of what we do in this course will involve feet, inches, meters, and millimeters.

EXERCISES: (Round answers to two decimal places.)

1. Convert 155mm to inches. (Hint: 155mm = how many meters? Now convert to inches.)

2. How many feet are in 155mm? (Hint: Convert the answer in #1 to feet.)

3. Convert 6 feet to meters. (Hint: How many inches in 6 feet? Convert this number to cm, and then convert that answer to meters.)

4. Convert 20 feet to meters.

5. How many inches long is a 120mm riding bow temple?

6. Convert the standard reading distance of 16 inches to centimeters.

7. My computer monitor is 30 inches away from my face. How many meters is this?

8. How many feet are there in a one-meter stick?

SINE, COSINE, TANGENT

The *sine* (pronounced like sign), *cosine* and *tangent* are *functions of angles*. They are abbreviated *sin*, *cos*, and *tan*. *These functions are used only when angles are involved.* If you wish to learn more about these functions than presented here, refer to a basic Trigonometry textbook in the library.

How you solve the equations containing angles depends on what type of calculator you have. If you do not have a calculator, or your calculator does not have these keys, use option **c** in each of the examples below. If you have a calculator with a key labeled "sin", perform the following test:

1. Turn the calculator on.
2. Press **30**.
3. Press the key labeled **sin**.
4. If the calculator says **0.5**, use option **a** in the examples below. If not:
5. Press **C** or **CE** or whatever clear is on the calculator.
6. Press **sin**.
7. Press **30**.
8. Press **=**.

9. If the calculator says **0.5**, use option **b** in the examples below. If neither of these methods works, look in the directions on how to change the calculator to degrees from radians, or ask someone for help.

When the angle is GIVEN and the sine of the angle is needed, either:

a. Enter the value of the angle in the calculator and then press the button that is labeled **sin**.

b. Press the button that is labeled **sin** on the calculator, enter the value of the angle, and then press the **equal** or **enter** button.

c. Turn to Appendix 4, **page 203-204**, look for the angle in column one or five, and read to the right across the line to the next column.

EXAMPLE:

1. sin 45 = ?

a. Enter **45**, press **sin**. If the calculator reads 0.707106..., this is the answer.

b. Press **sin**, enter **45**, press =. It should show 0.707106....

c. Turn to **page 203**. Find 45 at the bottom of the page in column one. Read to the right to the sine column, where it says 0.70711. This is the answer.

2. tan 61 = ?

a. Enter **61** in the calculator, press **tan**. It should show 1.804047...

b. Enter **tan, 61,** =. The display should show 1.804047...

c. On **page 203**, find 61 halfway down the fifth column. Read to the right to the last column, which is labeled tangent. The entry is 1.80405. This is the answer.

When the angle is NOT GIVEN, but the sine is given, either:

a. Enter the value in your calculator, press the **second** or **inverse** or **shift** button, and then press the **sin** button.

b. Press the **second** or **inverse** or **shift** button on your calculator, press the button that is labeled **sin**, enter the value, and then press the **equal** or **enter** button.

c. Turn to Appendix 4, **page 203-204**, look for the value in column two or six, and read back to the left one column to the angle.

You will be able to find only one of the keys: **inverse, second,** or **shift**.

EXAMPLE:

3. sin a = 0.24192. What is angle a?

a. Enter the value **0.24192** in your calculator. Press **second** (or **inverse** or **shift**), then **sin**. The calculator shows 13.999888.... This rounds to 14 degrees.

b. Press **second** (or **inverse** or **shift**), then **sin**, then enter the value **.24192**, then press =. The calculator shows 13.999888.... This rounds to 14 degrees.

c. Read down the column labeled sine on **page 203** until you come to 0.24192. Read to the left; the angle is 14 degrees.

4. cos β = 0.45. What is angle β?
   a. Enter the value **.45** in your calculator. Press **second** (or **inverse** or **shift**), then **cos**. The calculator shows 63.256.... This rounds to 63 degrees.
   b. Press **second** (or **inverse** or **shift**), then **cos**, then enter the value **0.45**, then press =. The calculator shows 63.256.... This rounds to 63 degrees.
   c. Read down the cosine column on **page 203** until you come to 0.45. It does not appear in the first cosine column; it is partway down the second cosine column. You will find 0.45399 and 0.43837. 0.45 is closer to 0.45399 than it is to 0.43837, so use the angle that corresponds to 0.45399, which is 63 degrees.

If you are using a calculator, to enter negative values, enter the value and press the +/- key, not the subtract (–) key.

EXERCISES: (Round answers 1-6 to five decimal places. Round angles to the nearest whole angle.)

1. sin 36 = ?   _____

2. cos 89 = ?   _____

3. tan 1 = ?   _____

4. sin 180 = ?   _____

5. cos 144 = ?   _____

6. tan 92 = ?   _____

7. sin a = 0.588. angle a = ?   _____

8. cos β = 0.588. angle β = ?   _____

9. tan δ = 0.36397. angle δ = ?   _____

10 tan θ = –0.36397. angle θ = ?   _____

11. cos α = –0.15643. angle α = ?   _____

12. sin a = 0.50. angle a = ?   _____
Note: If you are using the tables on pages 203-204, there are two angles with this sine.

13. $\sin^2 45$ = ?   _____
Note: This means, find the sine of 45 degrees, and then square the amount. Sin 45 = ?
Once you find this answer, press the x^2 key. On some calculators you must press shift before the x^2 key.

SECTION II: BASIC THEORY OF LIGHT

OVERVIEW OF THEORIES OF LIGHT

PARTICLE THEORIES OF LIGHT

In the 6th century BC the Greek philosopher and mathematician Pythagoras believed that light is composed of *particles* that are emitted by visible objects. In the 5th century BC Empedocles proposed that the eye is the source of vision; he believed that the eye sends out tentacle-like particles that grasp an object. Plato combined the theories, believing that objects emit particles and the eyes send out tentacles, and the two meet in midair.

Sir Isaac Newton (1642-1727) proposed the corpuscle theory of light. This theory states that light consists of a flow of very minute particles, or *corpuscles*, that are projected at a tremendous velocity from all light-emitting objects, and these particles are gathered by the eye. Newton demonstrated that white light is actually composed of all colors.

Max Planck (1858-1947) proposed the quantum theory of light. This theory states that energy is not radiated or absorbed in a continuous manner, but in definite units. These extremely small units are called *photons*. The unit of energy for the photon is a *quantum*.

WAVE THEORY OF LIGHT

In the 4th century BC, Aristotle proposed that light takes the form of *waves*, and only luminous objects emit these waves.

The wave theory was again proposed by Christian Huygens (1629-1695). His theory states that light is a *wave motion* taking place in a hypothetical material called the *ether*. Ether was proposed to fill all of space. Huygens concluded that light travels in waves similar to the wave motion in water. This motion is called transverse wave motion, because individual particles on the surface of the water move perpendicular to the direction of the wave movement.

Wave theory explains the bending of light around objects, called *diffraction*. Diffraction of light requires very minute measurements and very narrow slits, and it was not recognized until the late 1800s. Because of this apparent lack of diffraction, and because Newton's reputation was so strong, the wave theory was largely ignored until the 1800s.

James C. Maxwell (1831-1879) concluded that light is *electromagnetic* in nature and that it differs from other forms of electromagnetic radiation only in *wavelength*.

DUALISTIC NATURE

There is a single complete theory of light called Quantum Electro Dynamics, or the quantum theory of light and electricity. In the shorter wavelengths *(or higher frequencies)* of the electromagnetic spectrum, the particle model of the theory becomes the most

ELECTROMAGNETIC SPECTRUM

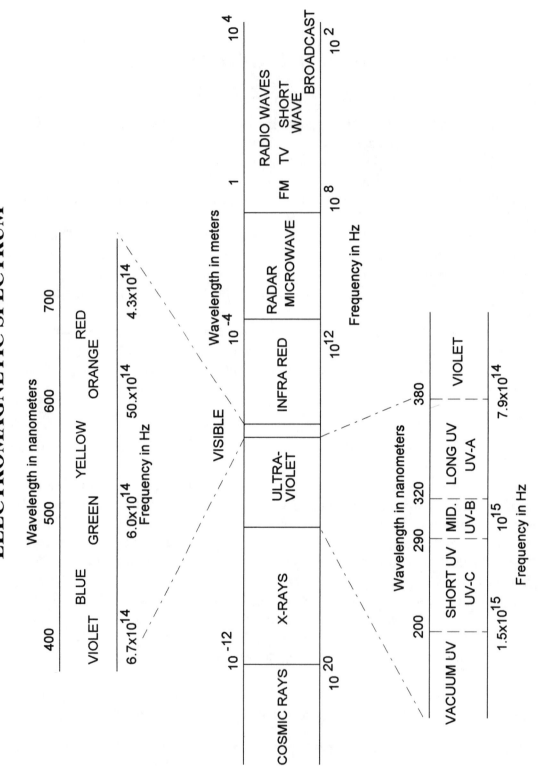

Adapted from *Clinical Optics, Second Edition,* by Fannin and Grosvenor, page 159.

important part of the theory and explains most observed properties; in the longer wavelengths, the wave model theory explains most properties. Visible light is in the intermediate portion where some properties are best explained with photons, and some with waves.

PROPERTIES OF WAVES

WAVELENGTH

Waves are described by their length. One *wavelength* is the distance from a point on one wave to the corresponding point on the next wave.

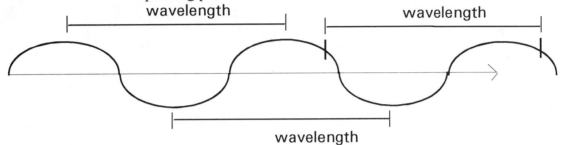

Waves of electromagnetic energy can be as long as miles, or as short as millionths of inches. Some waves can be measured in billionths of a meter. This unit of measurement is called a *nanometer*.

ONE NANOMETER = $1 \times 10^{-9}{}^{*}$ meters = 1×10^{-6} mm
    = 0.000,000,001 meter = 1/1,000,000,000 meters*

FREQUENCY

Frequency is the number of vibrations of a given wavelength in one second. In the electromagnetic spectrum, longer wavelengths vibrate fewer times, or, the shorter the wavelength, the higher the frequency. The unit of measurement for frequency is called the *hertz* **(Hz)**.

---

1 HERTZ = 1 COMPLETE WAVE PER SECOND.

Frequencies for visible light are large values and vary for each color of the spectrum.

RED LIGHT	$4.3 \times 10^{14}{}^{**}$ Hz
YELLOW LIGHT	5.4×10^{14} Hz
VIOLET LIGHT	7.5×10^{14} Hz

* A number $\times 10^{-9}$ means divide the number by 10 nine times, or move the decimal point nine places to the left.

** A number $\times 10^{14}$ means multiply the number by 10 fourteen times, or move the decimal point fourteen places to the right. Therefore, 4.3×10^{14} Hz = 430,000,000,000,000 waves/second.

VELOCITY

Velocity is the rate or speed at which light waves travel. In a vacuum, all waves in the electromagnetic spectrum travel at the same speed:

3×10^8 meters per second
(actually, 299,792,458 meters/second)
186,000 miles per second

Light travels slightly slower in air than in a vacuum, but not enough for us to be concerned with. As any given wave in the electromagnetic spectrum enters a material from air, it slows down. However, all wavelengths in the electromagnetic spectrum do not slow to the same speed in a particular material. White light is broken down into colors when it travels through a prism because the shorter blue waves slow more than the longer red waves. This is called *dispersion.* Dispersion was originally described by Newton in the late 1600s.

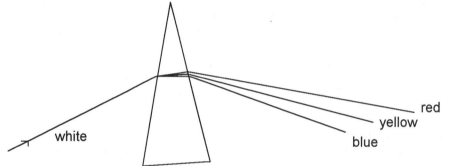

COLORS

In optics, we are concerned with ultraviolet, visible, and infrared waves.

	approximate WAVELENGTH (in mm or nm)	approximate FREQUENCY (in $\times 10^{14}$Hz)	
IR-C	3×10^{-3}mm - 1mm	0.003×10^{14} - 1×10^{14}Hz	
IR-B	1,400-3,000nm	1.0-2.1	lower energy,
IR-A	760-1,400	2.1-3.9	longer waves
red	660	4.5	fewer waves/sec
orange	610	4.9	
yellow	560	5.4	
green	510	5.9	
blue	460	6.5	
indigo	430	7.0	
violet	400	7.5	
UV-A	320-380	7.9-9.4	higher energy
UV-B	290-320	9.4-10.3	shorter waves
UV-C	200-290	10.3-15	more waves/sec

The infrared spectrum has waves that vary in wavelength from 0.001 m to 0.000,000,760 m. For IR waves, 300,000,000,000 to 390,000,000,000,000 go by every second.

The ultraviolet spectrum has waves that vary in wavelength from 0.000,000,200 m to 0.000,000,380 m. For UV waves, 1,500,000,000,000,000 to 790,000,000,000,000 go by every second.

> Regardless of wavelength or frequency, all electromagnetic
> waves travel at about 300,000,000 meters per second or
> 186,000 miles per second in a vacuum.

FACTS WE KNOW ABOUT LIGHT

1. Light spreads out from its source. It is *divergent* from the source. It has *negative vergence*.

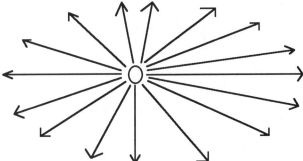

2. Light travels in straight lines. This is called the *rectilinear propagation of light.*

3. Light travels at a definite and constant speed in any given homogeneous medium or material.

> Visible light travels at:
> 186,000 miles per second in AIR
> 122,000 miles per second in CROWN GLASS
> 140,000 miles per second in WATER
> 124,000 miles per second in CR39

(The speed of light in a material is based on the speed of a yellow wave, λ = 588nm.)

WAVE FORMULA

The three properties of a wave are related by the formula

VELOCITY = FREQUENCY × WAVELENGTH

For any given color, only the frequency remains constant as the wave travels from one material to another.

$$v = f\lambda$$

or

$$f = v/\lambda$$

or

$$\lambda = v/f$$

where v = velocity of the wave: how far a peak travels in a unit of time,

f = frequency of the wave: how many peaks pass in a unit of time,

l.= wavelength of the wave: how far apart the peaks are.

EXAMPLE 1: What is the frequency in air of a ray of blue light that has a wavelength of 460nm, or 460×10^{-9}meters/wave? (In these exercises use $v = 3\times10^8$ meters/second for the velocity of light.)

$$f = v/\text{l} = (3 \times 10^8)/(460 \times 10^{-9}) = (3/460) \times 10^{+8+9}{}^* \text{ waves/second}$$
$$= 0.0065217 \times 10^{17}\text{Hz} = \mathbf{6.52 \times 10^{14}Hz.}$$

EXAMPLE 2: If a ray of red light has a wavelength of 660nm, what is its frequency in air?

$$f = v/\text{l} = (3 \times 10^8)/(660 \times 10^{-9}) = 0.00455 \times 10^{17} = \mathbf{4.55 \times 10^{14}Hz}$$

EXAMPLE 3: What does the wavelength of red light ($\lambda = 660$nm) change to when traveling from air to crown glass, where the wave travels at 1.97×10^8meters/sec, if its frequency is 4.55×10^{14}Hz?

$$\lambda = v/f = (1.97 \times 10^8)/(4.55\times10^{14}) = 0.433 \times 10^{8-14} = 0.433 \times 10^{-6}$$
$$= 433 \times 10^{-9} = \mathbf{433nm.}$$

WAVE FORMULA EXERCISES
(Round all answers to three digits.)

1. A ray of light has a wavelength of 588nm in a vacuum. What is its frequency?

2. A ray of light has a frequency of 5.10×10^{14}Hz. What is its wavelength in polycarbonate, where the ray travels at 1.89×10^8meters/sec?

3. What is the wavelength of the ray of light having a frequency of 5.10×10^{14}Hz while it travels through water, where the wave travels at 2.26×10^8meters/sec?

4. A ray of light has a frequency of 8.33×10^{14}Hz. What is the wavelength of this ray in a vacuum? What part of the electromagnetic spectrum is this ray?

VERGENCE

Divergent lines are lines that spread apart as if originating from a point. They have *negative vergence.* Sometimes divergent rays of light have to be projected back to a *virtual* or imaginary point or image. A virtual image cannot be projected onto a screen. It is *as if* the point of origin of the rays were there.

---

* Division by 10^{-9} is equal to multiplication times 10^9. To multiply 10^8 and 10^9, add the superscripts 8 and 9. Thus, $10^8/10^{-9} = 10^8\times10^9 = 10^{8+9} = 10^{17}$.

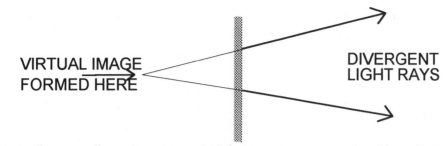

VIRTUAL IMAGE
FORMED HERE

DIVERGENT
LIGHT RAYS

Convergent lines are lines that come together to meet at a point (then diverge again as they continue on their path.) Convergent rays have *positive vergence.* Convergent rays of light will form a *real* image. A real image can be projected onto a screen.

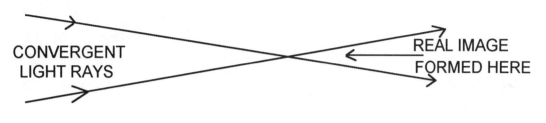

CONVERGENT
LIGHT RAYS

REAL IMAGE
FORMED HERE

Parallel lines are lines that never meet.

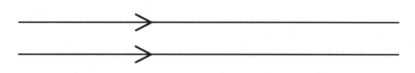

The farther light travels from its source, the less vergence it has, and the rays of light eventually become essentially parallel. Light rays originating from a distance of *20 feet* or *6 meters* or more are considered to be parallel. This is the definition of *optical infinity.*

PHOTONS, RAYS, PENCILS, AND BEAMS

A *photon* is a particle of light. It is the smallest amount of light possible. A *ray* is the path of a single photon of light from a single point on a light source.

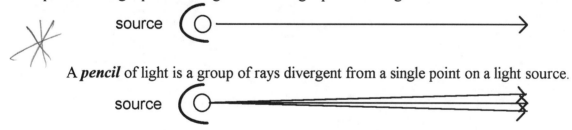

A *pencil* of light is a group of rays divergent from a single point on a light source.

source

A **beam** of light is composed of the group of pencils originating from all of the points on a light source.

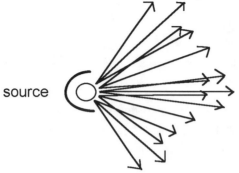

ILLUMINANCE

Illuminance varies with the square of the distance of the object from the light source:

$$E = \frac{I}{d^2}$$

where E is the intensity of the light on the object, in lux (lx) [or foot-candles],
I is the intensity of the light at the source, in lumens (lm),
d is the distance of the light source from the object in meters [or feet].

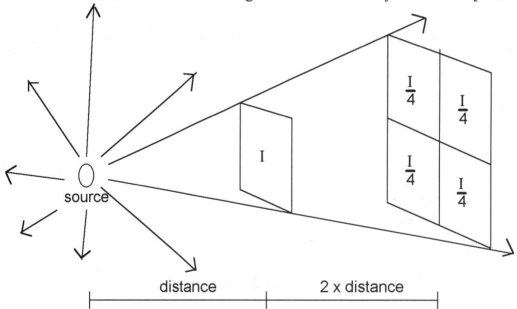

Light intensity used to be measured in foot-candles, which was the intensity of light generated by one candle on a one-square-foot surface one foot away. The formula using foot-candles is the same as above, but distance is measured in feet if intensity is in footcandles. Intensity is now more commonly measured in **lux.** One lux is one **lumen** (related to a candle) on a one square meter screen one meter away. One lux is approximately 10 foot-candles. (Actually, one lux = 10.76 foot-candles.)

If a book is 1 meter from a 100 lumen source, the intensity of light falling on the book is $100/1^2 = 100$ lux. If the book is 2m from the 100 lumen source, the intensity of the light falling on the book is $100/2^2 = 100/4 = 25$ lux.

Illuminance is a measurement of how much light is incident on a surface. It *is not* a measurement of how bright the surface appears to the observer. If none of the incident light reflects off of the surface, the surface *appears* dark, regardless of the intensity of the illumination or the distance of the surface from the light source.

The unit *candela* refers to the intensity of yellow light of wavelength 555nm, which is the wavelength that our eyes are most sensitive to. The candela is abbreviated cd. A 60 watt bulb will typically give off 120,000 cd/m². Good reading intensity is about 1,400 cd/m².

The lumen is a measurement of power, while the candela is a measurement of intensity as it relates to the physiology of the eye.

ILLUMINANCE EXERCISES
(Round answers to whole numbers.)

1. A 1,000 lumen light source is 4 meters away from the center of a screen. The edge of the screen is 5 meters from the light source.

   a. What is the intensity of light falling on the center of the screen?

   b. What is the intensity of light falling on the edge of the screen?

2. A slitlamp has a 300,000 lumen light source. What intensity of light falls on the patient's eye when it is 30cm away from the source? What intensity of light falls on the eye when it is 40cm from the source?

ABSORPTION, REFLECTION, REFRACTION

Three things may happen when light meets an object:

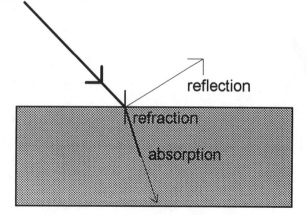

1. ABSORPTION

Absorption is what happens when a photon of light enters a material, but does not exit again. Absorption of photons in the electromagnetic spectrum may result in thermal, electrical, or chemical changes. These are all just different forms of energy. Dark colors absorb more than light colors. Visible and infrared waves are absorbed by most materials as heat; this is why we wear dark colors in the winter and light colors in the summer.

2. REFLECTION

Reflection occurs when a light ray is turned back into the incident material instead of traveling on into the new material. If the surface of the new material is relatively smooth, then any two rays that are reflected from the surface will continue to travel with the same relationship to each other that they originally had. In other words, the reflection changed the direction of the rays, but not their vergence with respect to each other. This is *regular* or *specular* reflection, and results in a surface that is interpreted as shiny. If the surface is not smooth, then the rays seem to reflect back in a random manner with respect to each other, and the result is *diffuse* reflection.

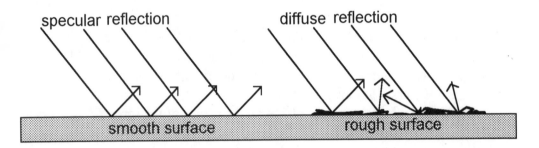

It is the light reflected by an object that gives it its color. An object appears to be black if it absorbs all of the wavelengths of the visible spectrum. An object appears to be white if it reflects diffusely all of the wavelengths of the visible spectrum. An object appears to be red if it reflects light from the red portion of the spectrum and absorbs all others.

3. REFRACTION

Refraction is the bending or change in direction of light when it passes from one transparent material to another transparent material of a different optical density.

FACTORS AFFECTING REFRACTION:

1. **The material itself.** Each material has a different optical density, which affects how much it slows a light ray down. So each material has a particular refracting ability.

2. **The obliquity of the incident light ray.** Light rays incident normal (meaning perpendicular) to a surface slow down, but do not change direction. Rays incident at any other angle will change direction, or be bent. The greater the angle at which the ray meets the surface, the more it changes direction, or is bent.

3. **The wavelength of the incident light ray.** Light rays with different wavelengths travel at different speeds in any particular material. Only in a vacuum do all wavelengths travel at the same speed.

LAW OF REFLECTION

When a ray of light is reflected from a surface, whether it is rough or smooth, the angle of reflection will equal the angle of incidence.

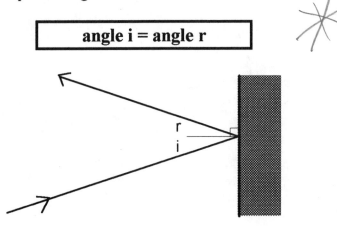

The angles of incidence and reflection are measured using the normal to the surface (which is the line perpendicular to the surface). For a smooth surface, because the angles are equal, the vergence of incident light is not changed. Two rays striking the surface at an angle to each other will leave the surface at the same angle to each other.

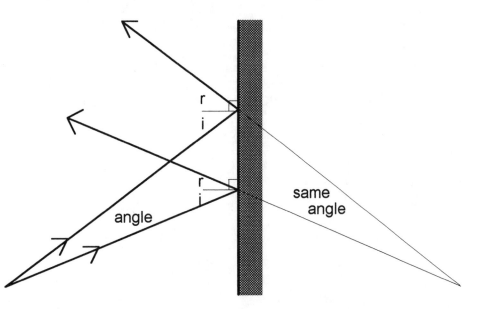

This is why an image in a flat mirror appears to be the same distance behind the mirror that the object is in front of the mirror. The formulas dealing with reflection from flat and curved surfaces will be discussed in Section VII, Image Formation.

LAWS OF REFRACTION

1. A ray of light striking a transparent surface **normal** (perpendicular) to the surface will not be bent, but the speed of the light will be changed because of the change in density of the material.

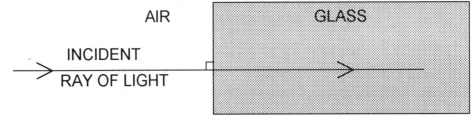

2. Light passing obliquely (at an angle other than perpendicular) from a material of *lesser* density to a material of *greater* density will be bent *toward* the normal.

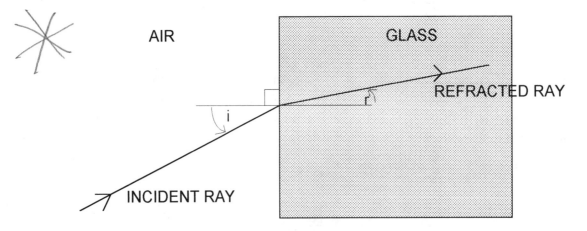

3. Light passing obliquely from a material of *greater* density to a material of *lesser* density will be bent *away* from the normal.

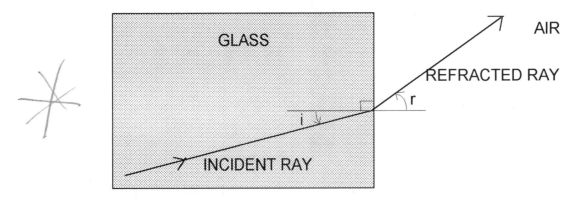

The angle between the light ray and the normal to the surface between the two materials is called the **angle of incidence,** or **i**. The angle at which the ray emerges into the second material is the **angle of refraction** or **r**. The angle between the path of the refracted ray and the path the ray would have taken if it had not bent is the **angle of deviation**, or δ (delta).

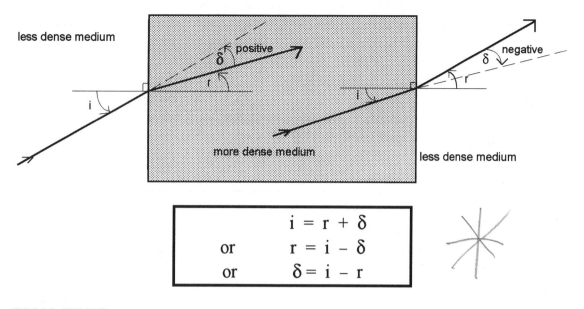

$$i = r + \delta$$
or $$r = i - \delta$$
or $$\delta = i - r$$

EXAMPLES:

1. If the angle of incidence is 20 degrees, and the angle of refraction is 15 degrees, then by how much is the ray deviated?

    $\delta = i - r = 20 - 15 = 5$ degrees.

2. If the ray is deviated by −18 degrees from its original path, and the angle of incidence is 48 degrees, then what is the angle of refraction?

    $r = i - \delta = 48 - (-18) = 48 + 18 = 66$ degrees.

3. If the angle of deviation is 16 degrees, and the angle of refraction is 40 degrees, then what is the angle of incidence?

    $i = r + \delta = 40 + 16 = 56$ degrees.

ANGLE EXERCISES

1. If a ray of light traveling through air is incident on a plane surface at 20 degrees and is deviated 5 degrees from its original path by the new material, what is the angle of refraction?

2. If a ray of light entering a plane glass block from air is deviated from its path by 10 degrees and its angle of refraction is 5 degrees, what was the angle of incidence of the ray of light?

3. If a ray of light leaving a material and traveling into air is incident on the surface at 15 degrees and it is refracted through an angle of 33 degrees, what is the angle of deviation? (Why is this angle negative?)

4. If a ray of light traveling from glass into air has an angle of incidence of 25 degrees and is deviated -4 degrees, what is its angle of refraction?

INDEX OF REFRACTION

The index of refraction of a transparent material is a ratio that compares the speed of light in a vacuum to the speed of light as it moves through the material. The speed of light in a vacuum is 186,000 miles per second, or 3×10^8 meters per second. Although a ray of light will be slowed when it enters air from a vacuum, it is not slowed enough to affect our calculations, so the speed of light is approximated at 186,000 miles/sec and 3×10^8 meters/sec in either air or vacuum. (We actually use the speed of a yellow wave, $\lambda = 588$nm, for the index of refraction.)

The small letter n is the symbol for index of refraction in this book. Some books use the Greek letter mu (μ) for this.

$$n = \frac{\text{SPEED OF LIGHT IN AIR}}{\text{SPEED OF LIGHT IN A MATERIAL}}$$

Alternatively,

$$\text{SPEED OF LIGHT IN A MATERIAL} = \frac{\text{SPEED OF LIGHT IN AIR}}{n}$$

The amount of refraction or bending of light by a material is dependent on the speed of light through the material. The more the ray is slowed, the more it is bent or refracted.

The higher the index of refraction, the slower the light travels through the material, and the more the ray is bent. This is why a higher index lens is thinner than a lower index lens of the same power. The material slows the light more, so the curve on the lens bends the light more than the same curve would do on a lower index lens.

Here are the indices for some common ophthalmic materials:

```
AIR = 1.00
WATER = 1.33
CR39 = 1.498 OR 1.50
TOOLS IN MOST LABS ARE CALIBRATED TO 1.53
CROWN GLASS = 1.523
POLYCARBONATE = 1.586
BARIUM GLASS ≈ 1.60 (depending on content)
FLINT GLASS ≈ 1.70 (depending on content)
High index plastics: available in many indices.
High index glass: now available over 1.70.
Cornea of the eye = 1.37 (average)
Lens of the eye = 1.42 (average)
Aqueous, vitreous and tear film = 1.34 (average)
```

INDEX OF REFRACTION EXERCISES

Using 186,000 miles/second for the speed of light in the following exercises, round the indices to two decimal places. (Mathematically, only one decimal place is justified.)

1. If light has a speed of 118,000mps in a transparent material, what is the index of refraction of that material?

2. What is the refractive index of a material if the speed of light passing through it is 109,000mps?

3. How fast will light travel through a material of refractive index 1.53? (Round to thousands.)

SNELL'S LAW

When a ray of light travels from one material, the ***incident*** material, to another material, the ***refracting*** material, the direction of the ray will be deviated according to Snell's law:

$$\boxed{n_i \sin i = n_r \sin r}$$

where n_i = the index of refraction of the incident material,

n_r = the index of refraction of the refracting material,

i = the angle that the incident light ray makes with the normal (perpendicular) to the surface,

r = the angle that the refracted light ray makes with the normal (perpendicular) to the surface.

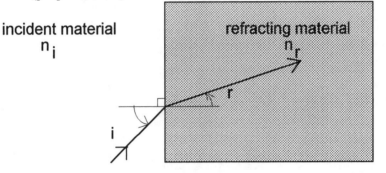

EXAMPLES:

1. If a ray of light travels from air into crown glass, with an angle of incidence of 30 degrees, what will the angle of refraction be? What is the angle of deviation?

$n_i = 1$	$n_i \sin i = n_r \sin r$
$n_r = 1.523$	$(1)(\sin 30) = (1.523)(\sin r)$
$i = 30$	$0.5 = (1.523)(\sin r)$
$r = ?$	$\sin r = (0.5)/(1.523)$
$\delta = ?$	$\sin r = 0.32830$
	r = 19 degrees
	$\delta = i - r = 30 - 19 =$ **11 degrees**

2. If a ray of light travels from crown glass into air with an angle of incidence of 30 degrees, what will the angle of refraction be? What is the angle of deviation?

$n_i = 1.523$ $n_i \sin i = n_r \sin r$

$n_r = 1$ $(1.523)(\sin 30) = (1)(\sin r)$

$i = 30$ $(1.523)(0.5) = \sin r$

$r = ?$ $\sin r = 0.7615$

$\delta = ?$ **r = 50 degrees**

$$\delta = i - r = 30 - 50 = \textbf{-20 degrees}$$

Note: Because the ray is going from a more dense material to a less dense material, the angle of refraction is greater than the angle of incidence, and the deviation is negative. (Look at the right side of the diagram on page 21)

3. If a ray of light travels from an unknown material into air with an angle of refraction of 20 degrees and an angle of incidence of 13 degrees, what is the index of the material?

$n_i = ?$ $n_i \sin i = n_r \sin r$

$n_r = 1$ $(n_i)(\sin 13) = (1)(\sin 20)$

$i = 13$ $(n_i)(0.22495) = 0.34202$

$r = 20$ $n_i = (0.34202) / (0.22495)$

$n_i = 1.52$

SNELL'S LAW EXERCISES

(Round angles to whole angles.)

1. If a ray of light travels from crown glass (n=1.523) into air with an angle of incidence of 35 degrees, what will the angle of refraction be?

2. If a ray of light travels from air into CR39 (n=1.498) with an angle of incidence of 28 degrees, what will the angle of refraction be?

3. If a ray of light travels from CR39 (n=1.498) into air and emerges into the air with an angle of 45, what was the angle of incidence?

CRITICAL ANGLE

When light travels from a more dense material to a less dense material at just the right oblique angle, it is possible for the ray to emerge parallel to the surface of the refracting material. In this case the angle of refraction, r, is 90°, and sin r = 1. The angle of incidence necessary for this to occur will satisfy the equation $n_i \sin i = n_r$, or

$$\sin i = n_r / n_i$$

When the ray is traveling into air, this reduces to $n_i \sin i = 1$, or

$$\sin i = 1 / n$$

The angle i which satisfies the equation is the *critical angle* of the **material of index n in air.** A ray that is incident at an angle greater than the critical angle will be reflected back into the incident material, or be reflected internally. This is *total internal reflection*.

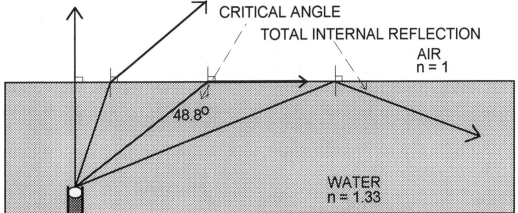

EXAMPLE 1: What is the critical angle in air of water, n = 1.33?
Sin i = 1/n = 1/1.33 = 0.75188. This gives an angle of 48.8° or 49°. This means that, if a beam of light traveling from water to air is at an angle to the surface that is greater than 49°, then the beam is reflected back into the water.

EXAMPLE 2: What is the critical angle in air of a diamond with n = 2.42?
Sin i = 1/2.42 = 0.41322; i = 24.
A ray attempting to leave a diamond, n = 2.42, will reflect back into the diamond if the angle of incidence is greater than 24°.

EXAMPLE 3: What is the critical angle of CR39 in air?
sin i = 1/n = 1/1.498 = 0.66756; i = 42 degrees

CRITICAL ANGLE EXERCISES
(Round angles to whole numbers)

1. What is the critical angle of flint glass in air? (n = 1.70)

2. What happens to a ray of light leaving CR39 (n = 1.498) and entering air if the angle of incidence is: (Use Snell's law.)
    a. 15 degrees?

    b. 25 degrees?

    c. 35 degrees?

    d. 45 degrees?
    (**Note**: When you try to find i for sin i = 1.05925, the calculator indicates an error. This is because 45° is greater than the critical angle for CR39, and indicates that the rays will all be reflected internally.)
    e. 55 degrees?

3. What is the critical angle of a diamond (n = 2.42) which is immersed in water?

DISPERSION AND ABBE NUMBER

Visible light travels at about 186,000 miles/second in a vacuum. So do X-rays, radio waves, and everything else in the electromagnetic spectrum. When a ray or wave enters any material traveling from a vacuum, it slows down. However, different waves will be slowed different amounts. An X-ray will not travel at the same speed in crown glass, for example, as a ray from the infrared spectrum.

The same is true of the different wavelengths in the visible spectrum. Red waves of wavelength 660nm will travel at a different speed in crown glass than blue waves of wavelength 460nm. The index of refraction is measured for yellow light, wavelength 588nm. However, the index of refraction for any particular material actually varies, depending on the wavelength of the light ray.

For all of our glasses lens materials, shorter waves are slowed more than longer waves. Therefore, when white light (made up of all colors) passes through a lens, the blue waves are refracted more than the red waves, and the light is broken down into its component colors. This is *dispersion*. It causes *chromatic aberrations.* The image formed by the blue rays is a different distance from the lens than the image formed by the red rays, resulting in fringes of color around the images seen through the lens. The ability of a material to break white light into its component colors is measured using the *Abbe number* of the material. To compute the Abbe number, we need to know the index of refraction for several different wavelengths. The standard in the United States is to use $\lambda = 588$nm for yellow, $\lambda = 486$ for blue, and $\lambda = 656$ for red.

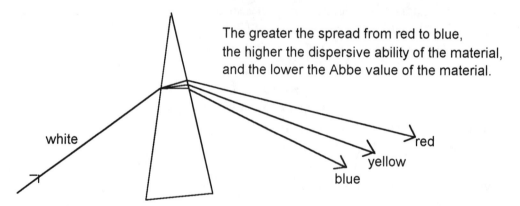

The greater the spread from red to blue, the higher the dispersive ability of the material, and the lower the Abbe value of the material.

The formula for the Abbe number is

$$\frac{n_{yellow} - 1}{n_{blue} - n_{red}}$$

The Abbe number is also called the *V-value*, or the *nu value,* or the *constringence.* The Abbe number is the inverse of the *dispersive value* of the material.

EXAMPLE: For a particular crown glass, n_{yellow} = 1.5230, n_{blue} = 1.5293, and n_{red} = 1.5204.* The Abbe number for this glass is

$$\frac{1.5230 - 1}{1.5293 - 1.5204} = \frac{0.5230}{0.0089} = 58.76 = 59$$

In this case, the n's for red and blue are relatively close together, so the denominator is relatively small and the Abbe number is relatively large. The higher the Abbe number, the lower the dispersive value for the material and the less the chromatic aberration of the lens.

The Abbe numbers for some common ophthalmic materials:

Crown glass	59-61
CR39	56-58
Barium crown	low 50s
Flint	low 30s
Polycarbonate	29-31

ABBE NUMBER EXERCISE

For a particular flint glass, n_{yellow} = 1.7200, n_{blue} = 1.7378, and n_{red} = 1.7130.* What is the Abbe number of the material? (Round to the nearest whole number.) What is the index of refraction of the material?

Note: The denominator of this fraction is relatively large compared to the denominator of the Abbe value for crown glass. Because the n's for red and blue are much further apart in this flint glass, the chromatic aberration for this material is much greater than for crown glass and the Abbe value for the material is smaller than the value for crown glass.

---

* The values for n are taken from Meyer-Arendt, *Introduction to Classical and Modern Optics,* page 19.

SECTION III: LENSES

REFRACTION THROUGH A LENS

A *lens* is composed of a transparent material with two polished surfaces, at least one of which is curved. A lens changes the *vergence* of the incident light.

Parallel rays of light are said to have *no vergence* or *zero vergence*. Rays of light traveling toward each other are *converging*, or have *positive vergence*. Rays of light traveling away from each other are *diverging*, or have *negative vergence*. By convention, a distance measured in the direction of travel of the light ray will be positive, and a distance measured opposite the direction of travel of the light ray will be negative.

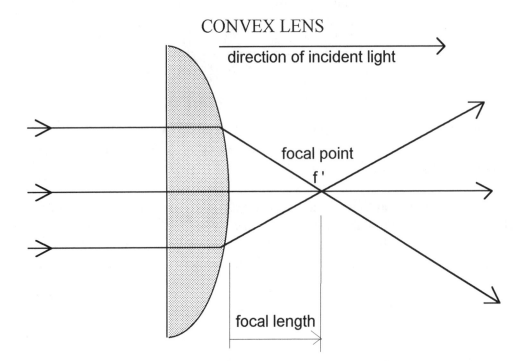

The lens pictured here is changing the vergence of the incident rays of light. Incident rays with zero vergence (parallel rays) are changed by this lens to rays with positive vergence (converging rays). If the incident rays were already converging, then they would emerge with higher positive vergence. If the incident rays had negative vergence, they would emerge with either less negative vergence, zero vergence, or positive vergence. The change in vergence caused by the lens is a result of the index of refraction of the lens material and the curvature of the two lens surfaces.

Because this lens increases the vergence of the rays, it is a converging lens, has a positive focal length, and is a positive lens. The *focal point* of the lens (actually the secondary focal point) is the point where the parallel incident rays cross. The focal point is considered a *real* focal point because the rays *actually cross there*. This focal length is *positive* because the measurement is from the lens to the secondary focal point, which is in the direction of travel of the rays of light.

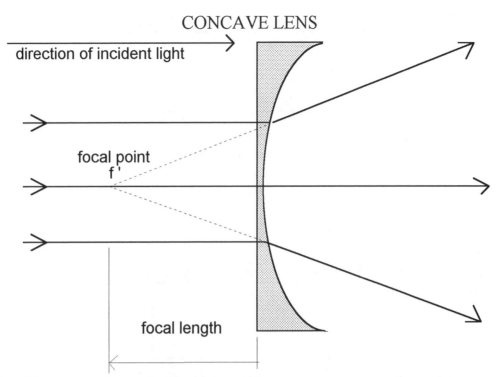

CONCAVE LENS

direction of incident light

focal point
f '

focal length

For this concave lens, incident rays with zero vergence are changed to rays with negative vergence; they are now diverging rays. If the incident rays were already diverging, then they would emerge with higher negative vergence. If the incident rays had positive vergence, they would emerge with either less positive vergence, zero vergence, or negative vergence. The change in vergence caused by the lens is a result of the index of refraction of the lens material and the curvature of the two lens surfaces.

Because this lens increases the divergence of the rays, it is a diverging lens, has a negative focal length, and is a negative lens. The **focal point** of the lens (actually the secondary focal point) is the point from which the rays would have emerged in order to have the observed amount of divergence. The focal point is considered a **virtual focal point** because the rays *did not actually emerge from there*. This focal length is **negative** because the measurement is from the lens to the secondary focal point, which is opposite to the direction of travel of the rays of light.

FOCAL LENGTH FORMULA

The unit of measurement of the refractive power of a lens or a surface is the **Diopter**. The diopter was introduced by a French ophthalmologist, Monoyer, in 1872. The capital letter D stands for diopter in our optical formulas. When the lens is in air, the power of the lens in diopters is equal to the reciprocal of the focal length of the lens in meters.

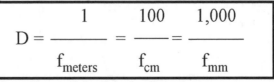

$$D = \frac{1}{f_{meters}} = \frac{100}{f_{cm}} = \frac{1,000}{f_{mm}}$$

where   D is the power of the lens in diopters
             f is the focal length of the lens in meters, cm, or mm.

When the focal length is given in inches the formula becomes:

$$D = \frac{39.37}{f_{inches}} \approx \frac{40}{f_{inches}}$$

EXAMPLE 1: What is the dioptric power of a lens that has a focal length of +0.5m?
$$D = 1/f = 1/0.5 = +2.00D.$$

EXAMPLE 2: What is the dioptric power of a lens that brings parallel rays of light to a point focus 16 inches from the lens?
$$D = 40/f = 40/16 = +2.50D.$$

When a lens is in a material other than air, the formula becomes

$$D = \frac{n}{f_{meters}}$$

or

$$f_{meters} = \frac{n}{D}$$

where n is the index of the material surrounding the lens.

EXAMPLE 3: A lens has a focal length of 20cm when it is in water. What is the dioptric power of the lens? (n = 1.33)
$$D = 1.33/0.20 = +6.65D$$

FOCAL LENGTH FORMULA EXERCISES

1. What is the dioptric power of a lens that has a focal length of +5cm?

2. What is the focal length in inches of a lens of power +4.00D?

3. What is the focal length of a −5.00D lens?

4. The eye contains a plus lens, which is able to change shape. When the eye is at rest,

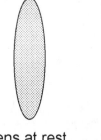

lens at rest

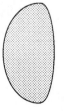

lens accommodating

the lens has an approximate power of +20D. When the lens accommodates, the shape of the lens changes, adding plus power. If the eye at rest focuses at infinity, and if it can accommodate to focus on this page, which is probably about 40cm away, then the lens must add enough plus power to bring the focus from infinity to 40cm. How much plus power must it *add* to accommodate for reading?

5. A young child can focus from infinity to 10cm away. How much plus power must this child's crystalline lens be able to add during accommodation for the distance of 10cm?

6. A lens has a focal length of 8 inches. What is its dioptric power?

DIOPTERS

In practice, diopters are expressed in increments of one-eighth of a diopter. All eighths are truncated to two decimal places. For example, one-eighth is 0.125, but this is truncated (changed) to 0.12.

```
STANDARD DIOPTRIC INCREMENTS:
        0.12D
        0.25D
        0.37D
        0.50D
        0.62D
        0.75D
        0.87D
        0.00D
```

A lens or surface will also have a sign to show whether it is a converging (+) or a diverging (−) lens or surface.

In the exercises in this book, if we are referring to a lens that might actually be ordered or made, we will change the dioptric values to one of these decimal increments. In many calculations, the end result will be an effective power, and then we will not change the answer to eighths because the result of the exercise would not necessarily be a lens that a person would wear. (See exercises, page 4.)

LENS SURFACES

There are three types of surface used in lens design. These are *plane*, *convex*, and *concave*.

PLANE SURFACE

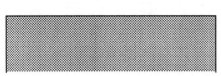

1. Flat surface.
2. Does not change the vergence of incident light
3. No (zero) power.
4. Abbreviated pl.

CONCAVE SURFACE

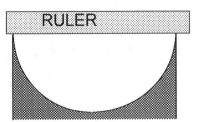

1. Hollow surface.
2. A flat edge placed on the surface does not rock, since it touches at two places.
3. Decreases the vergence of incident light; diverges light rays.
4. Has minus power.

CONVEX SURFACE

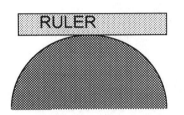

1. Bulging surface.
2. A flat edge placed on the surface rocks, since it is only touching in one spot.
3. Increases vergence of incident light; converges light rays.
4. Has plus power.

LENS TYPES

Lens surfaces can be combined in different ways to give different lens types. Lenses are classified as being either *flat* or *bent*. They are also classified by their surface combinations.

A **bent** lens is a lens that has one convex surface and one concave surface.

PLANO POWER   MINUS POWER   PLUS POWER

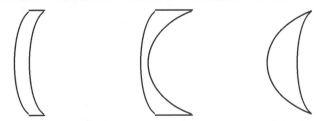

A **flat** lens is a lens that is not bent. It can have one flat surface combined with either one concave or one convex surface. It can have two concave surfaces, or it can have two convex surfaces.

EQUI-CONVEX   BI-CONVEX   PLANO-CONVEX

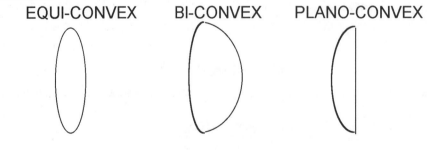

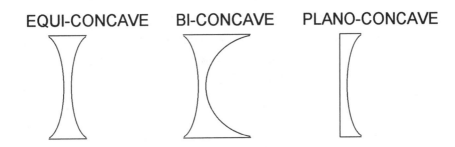

EQUI-CONCAVE   BI-CONCAVE   PLANO-CONCAVE

All of these lenses are examples of flat lens designs. If a lens does not have one convex surface and one concave surface, it is a flat design.

NOMINAL POWER FORMULA

The nominal power of a lens is the combined power of its front and back surfaces. We normally refer to the convex surface on a bent (or *meniscus*) lens as the front surface. The nominal power formula disregards the thickness of the lens and is sometimes referred to as the *thin lens formula.*

$$D_N = D_1 + D_2$$

or

$$D_1 = D_N - D_2$$

or

$$D_2 = D_N - D_1$$

where D_N is the nominal power of the lens in diopters,

D_1 is the front surface power in diopters,

D_2 is the back surface power in diopters.

Since this formula disregards the thickness of the lens, it is an approximation and should only be used for lens powers below +4.00D.

EXAMPLE 1: If the front surface power is +6.00D and the back surface power is −10.00D, then the lens has a nominal power of +6.00 + (−10.00) = −4.00D. Historically, a bent lens with a front surface power of +6.00D or a back surface power of −6.00D was called a *meniscus* lens. Now, we refer to *any* bent lens as a *meniscus* lens, and a bent lens with one surface of +/−6.00D as a *true meniscus* lens or a *Meniscus* lens.

EXAMPLE 2: A lens has a front surface power of +1.00D and a back surface power of −8.25D. What is its nominal power?
    $D_N = D_1 + D_2 = (+1.00) + (−8.25) = −7.25D$.

EXAMPLE 3: If a lens has a nominal power of +3.50 and a front surface of +9.25, what is its back surface power?
    $D_2 = D_N − D_1 = (+3.50) − (+9.25) = −5.75D$.

NOMINAL POWER AND LENS TYPES WORKSHEET
(Change to one-eighth diopter steps.)

Look at the following drawings and determine the power of each lens. Describe each lens stating whether is *bent* or *flat,* and name the lens type, such as *bi-convex* or *equi-concave.*

	NOMINAL POWER	BENT/ FLAT	LENS TYPE

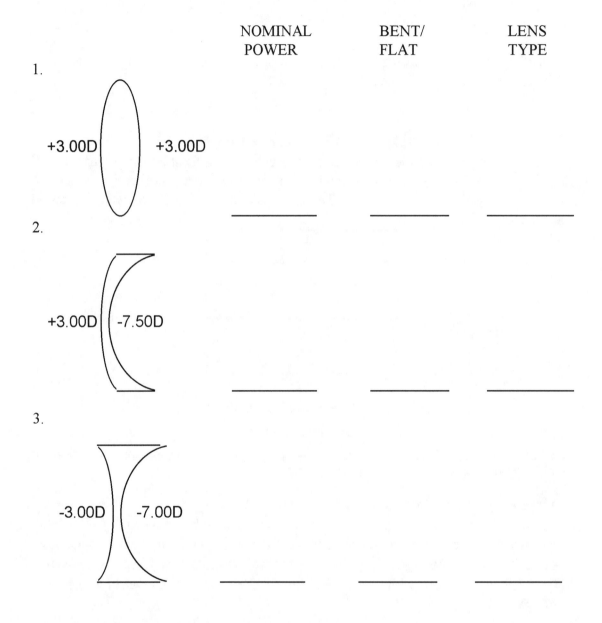

1.

+3.00D   +3.00D

_____   _____   _____

2.

+3.00D -7.50D

_____   _____   _____

3.

-3.00D   -7.00D

_____   _____   _____

4. What is the nominal power of an equi-convex lens where both surface powers are +2.37D?

5. What is the front surface power of a +4.00D lens if it has a back surface power of −3.62D?

6. What is the back surface power of a −3.00D lens if it has a front surface power of +2.25D?

7. What is the front surface power of a +3.75D lens if it has a back surface power of −1.25D? (This lens was historically called a ***periscopic*** lens. The first popular bent lens had a front surface power of +1.25D for all minus lenses and a back surface power of −1.25D for all plus lenses. This design was supplanted by the *true meniscus* lens discussed in example 1 on page 33.)

8. If I need a lens with an Rx of +3.00D, and I am given a lens blank with a front surface of +9.00, what power curve would I need to create on the back of the lens?

RADIUS OF CURVATURE

A surface must be curved for it to alter the vergence of the light striking it. A surface with a long radius of curvature will be a relatively flat surface, so the change in vergence will be small. A surface with a short radius of curvature will have a relatively steep surface, so the change in vergence will be large.

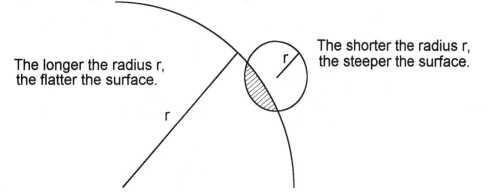

The longer the radius r, the flatter the surface.

The shorter the radius r, the steeper the surface.

The amount of vergence change caused by a lens surface will also depend on the refractive index of the material it is made of. The dioptric power of a lens surface can be determined using the surface power formula.

SURFACE POWER FORMULA

$$D = \frac{n_r - n_i}{r}$$

where   D is the power of the surface in diopters,

            n_r is the refractive index of the refracting side of the surface,

            n_i is the refractive index of the incident side of the surface,

            r is the radius of curvature of the surface in meters.

For our purposes air is usually on one side of the surface. Air has a refractive index of 1. Therefore, the formula is more often written as:

$$D = \frac{n - 1}{r}$$

We are going to ignore whether the light is entering or leaving the lens when it is refracted by this surface. Using $1 - n$ for the numerator when the light leaves a lens surface (traveling back into air) changes the sign of the resulting surface power, and requires that we discuss the sign of r. Instead, for now we are going to take care of the sign when we combine two surfaces to form a lens. We will discuss the sign of r in Section VII.

EXAMPLE 1: What is the dioptric power of a crown glass (n = 1.523) surface with a radius of curvature of 35cm? (Note: The radius in the formula is in meters, so 35cm = 0.35m.)

$$D = (1.523 - 1) / (0.35) = 1.49D$$

The surface power formula can be rearranged to find the radius of curvature of a surface:

$$r = \frac{n - 1}{D}$$

EXAMPLE 2: What is the radius of curvature in millimeters of a +5.00D surface made of crown glass? (n = 1.523)

$D = +5.00D$

$n = 1.523$ $\qquad r = (1.523 - 1) / (5) = 0.1046m = 104.6mm$

THE LENSMAKER'S EQUATION

The nominal power of a lens is given by the formula $D_N = D_1 + D_2$. This formula does not take into account the lens material or its curvature. A lensmaker makes a lens by producing curves on the front and back surfaces of the lens. The lensmaker used to determine the curves needed by using the lensmaker's equation.

$$D = {}^+/_- \frac{n - 1}{r_1} {}^+/_- \frac{n - 1}{r_2}$$

where D is the power of the lens in diopters,
n is the refractive index of the lens material,
r_1 is the radius of curvature of the front surface in meters,
r_2 is the radius of curvature of the back surface in meters.

Note: When using the lensmaker's equation,

         + is used when the surface is convex, and

         − is used when the surface is concave.

EXAMPLE: What is the power of a crown glass (n = 1.523) meniscus lens made with a front surface curve of 10cm and an ocular or back surface curve of radius 20cm?

D = ?

n = 1.523

r_1 = 10cm = 0.1m

r_2 = 20cm = 0.2m

$$D = +\frac{1.523 - 1}{0.1} - \frac{1.523 - 1}{0.2}$$

$$D = +5.23 - 2.62 = +2.61D, \text{ which changes to } +\textbf{2.62D}.$$

Note: The signs reflect that the front surface of a *meniscus* lens is convex and the back surface is concave.

There are several different sign conventions in use. For now we will consider the result of each surface calculation to be negative if the surface is concave, and positive if the surface is convex. We will explore the signs further in Section VII when we discuss thick lenses.

LENSMAKER'S EQUATION EXERCISES
(Change dioptric powers to the nearest one-eighth diopter.)

1. What is the dioptric power of a crown glass (n = 1.523) bi-concave lens with radii of curvature of 247mm and 149mm ?

2. What is the dioptric power of a meniscus CR39 (n = 1.498) lens which has a front surface curve of radius 40cm and a back surface curve of radius 16cm? (Do you remember what the old name for this style lens was?)

3. If a high-index lens with an index of refraction of 1.60 has a convex surface made on a tool with a radius of curvature of 8cm and a concave surface made on a tool with a radius of curvature of 15cm, what is the resulting power of the lens? What would the lens power have been if the material had been CR39? (n = 1.498)

CYLINDERS, COMPOUND LENSES

The surfaces that we have been talking about have been spherical surfaces. Every point on a spherical surface is an equal distance from a particular point called the center of the sphere. This distance is the radius of curvature of the surface.

Now consider lenses made with one or more surfaces that do not have a single center of curvature. Consider what a football looks like:

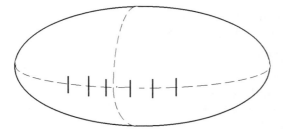

If you slice this surface in half horizontally, you see one curve.

If you slice the surface in half vertically, you see a much steeper curve.

This is a **toric surface**. If a donut lying flat on a surface is cut horizontally, the result is circles. If the donut is cut vertically, the result is circles. However, the horizontal circles are different size circles from the vertical circles, so the horizontal curvature is different from the vertical curvature. Looking at the surface of the donut lying flat on a table, or looking at the football pictured above, the **horizontal meridian** or direction is less curved than the **vertical meridian** or direction.

A toric surface is considered to be a spherical design, even though the surface is not a cut off of a sphere.

Now consider a **cylindrical surface**. A can is a cylinder: in this diagram the can has straight sides horizontally, round sides vertically.

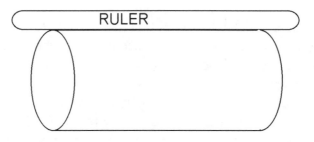

A ruler does not rock when placed along one direction, or meridian, of the surface. Therefore, a cylindrical surface is one with no power in one direction, maximum power 90 degrees away. The direction having no curvature is referred to as the **axis of the cylinder**. The can pictured here has a horizontal axis.

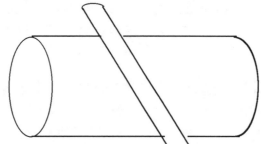

Placed in a different direction, or meridian, the ruler does rock. It rocks the most 90 degrees away from the axis of the cylinder.

A **compound lens**, or a **sphero-cylindrical lens,** is a lens with at least one (usually only one) toric surface. It can be thought of as a spherical lens sandwiched with a cylindrical lens having no power in one direction and the cylinder power in the other direction.

LENS MERIDIANS

Look at the diagrams of some lenses seen from the front and from the side. In each lens, there is a place where the lens is the thickest, and a place where it is the thinnest. In plus lenses, the thickest place is called the optical center of the lens. In a minus lens, the thinnest place is called the optical center of the lens. In each case, the optical center of the lens is the point on the lens surface where a ray of light will pass through the lens without changing directions. This occurs because, at this one point, the sides of the lens are parallel to each other.

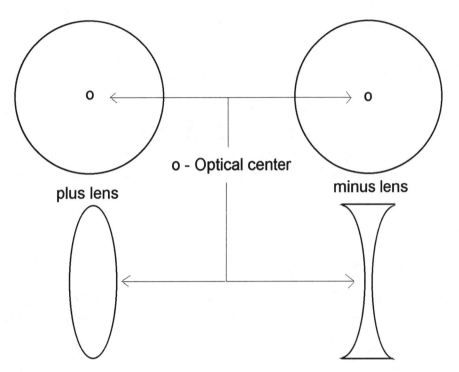

o - Optical center

plus lens   minus lens

An imaginary line on the lens surface that goes from one edge of the lens to the other edge, passing through the optical center of the lens, is called a meridian. Drawing meridians is like cutting the lens up into pie wedges. A meridian can be in any direction on the lens.

This meridian runs from 90 to 270 degrees.

This meridian is at 60 degrees, and runs to 240 degrees.

This meridian is at 30 degrees, and runs to 210 degrees.

This meridian goes from 0 to 180 degrees on a circle.

This meridian goes from 135 to 315 degrees.

When facing a person wearing glasses, the meridians run counterclockwise from the right side to the left side. For now, ignore the bottom of the lens.

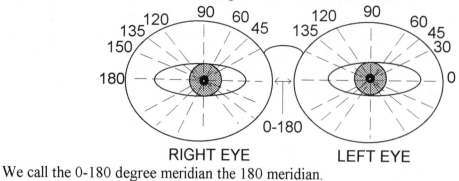

RIGHT EYE   LEFT EYE

We call the 0-180 degree meridian the 180 meridian.

OPTICAL CROSS

An optical cross is a graphical representation of the power of a lens, showing the power in the two major meridians on the lens. On a lens the two major meridians are always 90 degrees apart.

1. A SPHERE

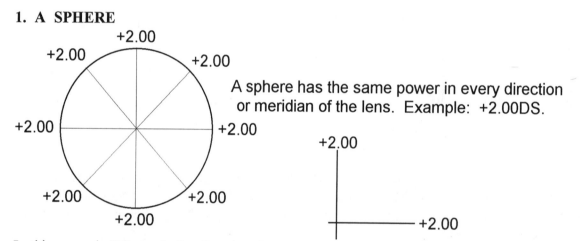

A sphere has the same power in every direction or meridian of the lens. Example: +2.00DS.

In this example DS stands for diopter sphere.

2. A CYLINDER

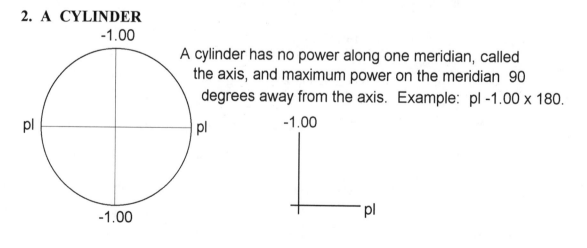

A cylinder has no power along one meridian, called the axis, and maximum power on the meridian 90 degrees away from the axis. Example: pl -1.00 x 180.

In this example, pl is the *sphere power*, −1.00 is the *amount of the cylinder,* and 180 is the *axis of the sphere*, also called the *axis of the prescription.*

3. A TORIC LENS

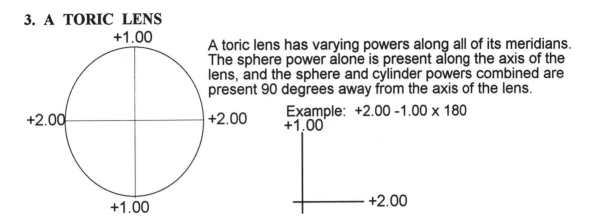

A toric lens has varying powers along all of its meridians. The sphere power alone is present along the axis of the lens, and the sphere and cylinder powers combined are present 90 degrees away from the axis of the lens.

Example: +2.00 -1.00 x 180

In this example, +2.00 is the *sphere power*, −1.00 is the *amount of the cylinder,* and 180 is the *axis of the sphere*, also called the *axis of the prescription.* This is also called a *sphero-cylindrical* lens or a *compound lens.*

PUTTING THE Rx ON THE OPTICAL CROSS

EXAMPLE: −1.50 +1.00 × 045

1.   Draw two lines 90 degrees from each other. They can be in the approximate orientation of the axis of the Rx, or they can be horizontal and vertical.

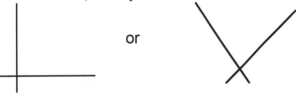

or

2.   Label the axis. Put the axis of the Rx on the end of one line. Add or subtract 90 from the axis, and put this number on the other line. The degree used must be between 0 and 180. Therefore, to find the second meridian, if the axis is 90 or less, add 90; if the axis is greater than 90, subtract 90.

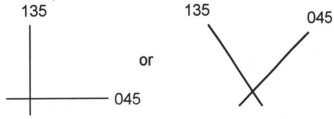

or

3. Put the sphere power on the axis line, since the sphere power alone is present along the axis of the prescription.

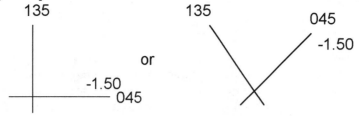

4. Add the sphere and cylinder powers together, and put the resulting total power on the line 90 degrees away from the axis of the prescription.

$$(-1.50) + (+1.00) = -0.50$$

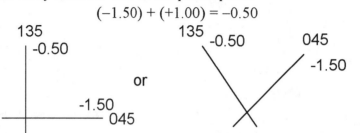

OPTICAL CROSS EXERCISES

Put the following prescriptions on an optical cross.

1. +3.50D

2. −1.00 −1.00 x180

3. +0.50 −2.00 x030

4. −1.00 +1.00 x080

5. −6.50 −0.50 x022

6. +4.25 − 1.75 x136

TAKING THE Rx OFF THE OPTICAL CROSS

There are three ways that a prescription can be written, so there are three ways in which it can be taken off the optical cross.

　　1. Minus cylinder form
　　2. Plus cylinder form
　　3. Cross cylinder form

1. MINUS CYLINDER FORM

Using the optical cross illustrated below:

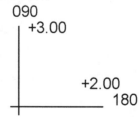

1. Sphere power: Take the most plus or the least minus power on the optical
   cross as the sphere power: +3.00D
2. Axis: The meridian of the power selected for the sphere will be the axis for the
   Rx: x090
3. Cylinder power: The *difference* between the powers in the two meridians gives
   the cylinder power. The cylinder power is found by subtracting the sphere
   power from the power on the other meridian: the power not used in step 1
   minus the power used. +2.00 − (+3.00) = −1.00D

The Rx is +3.00 −1.00 x090.

2. PLUS CYLINDER FORM

Using the same optical cross illustrated below:

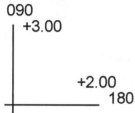

1. Sphere power: Take the least plus or the most minus power on the optical
   cross as the sphere power: +2.00D
2. Axis: The meridian of the power selected for the sphere will be the axis for the
   Rx: x180
3. Cylinder power: The *difference* between the powers in the two meridians gives
   the cylinder power. This is found by subtracting the sphere power from the
   power on the other meridian: the power not used in step 1 minus the
   power used. +3.00 − (+2.00) = +1.00D

The Rx is +2.00 +1.00 x180

Note: The cylinder represents how far the second power is from the first power. In the
minus cylinder example the cylinder was the result of moving from +3.00 to +2.00. In the
plus cylinder example we moved from +2.00 to +3.00.

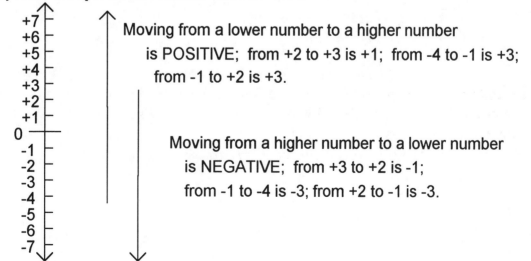

If you have been using a focimeter or lensometer, you will recognize the number line as the power drum. The technique and result are the same that you use when neutralizing glasses. You are determining the difference between the two dioptric values on the lens, and whether that difference is positive (going up on the power drum) or negative (going down on the power drum.)

EXAMPLE: Write the following Rx in plus cylinder form.

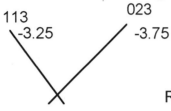

SPHERE: most minus: -3.75

CYLINDER: -3.25 - (-3.75) = +0.50

AXIS: where the sphere power is: 23

Rx in plus cylinder form: -3.75 +0.50 x 023

3. CROSS CYLINDER FORM

Using the optical cross illustrated below:

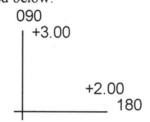

An alternative way to correct for a compound astigmatic error is to use two cylinders at right angles (90 degrees) to each other. The cross cylinders represent the powers on a toric surface. We will use this notation again when we study toric transposition. Remember, a cylinder has *plano power on its axis* and plus or minus power 90 degrees from its axis.

1. 1st cylinder: Select a power on one meridian, and assign it the axis from the other meridian: +3.00 x180
2. 2nd cylinder: Select the power on the other meridian, and assign it the axis from the first meridian: +2.00 x090

The Rx is +3.00 x180 ⊃ +2.00 x090.

The symbol ⊃ means *combined with*.

A cylinder has one plano side. An example of a plus cylinder is pl +5.00 x180. When referring to a true cylinder, we can write that same Rx as +5.00 x180, because the pl is *assumed* to be there. +5.00DC x180 is even more precise. Whenever an Rx is in the form *power* × *axis*, there is an assumed pl in front of the power. Thus, −3.50 × 125 means pl −3.50 ×125. This is why, in this notation, *the axis goes with the pl, not the power*.

EXAMPLE:

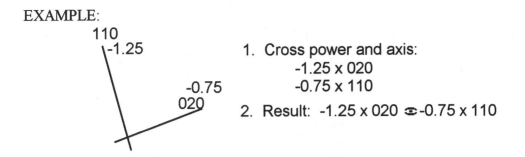

1. Cross power and axis:
    -1.25 x 020
    -0.75 x 110
2. Result: -1.25 x 020 ⊃ -0.75 x 110

Since we have now discussed cross cylinder form, we will discuss how to put a cross cylinder prescription on the optical cross.

   1. Place one of the axes on the optical cross diagram. Place the other cylinder power with this axis.
   2. Place the remaining cylinder power with the remaining axis.

EXAMPLE: Place the prescription +10.00 x023 ⊃ +7.50 x113 on the optical cross.

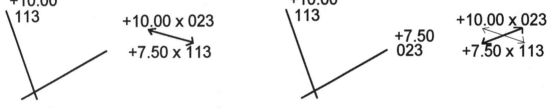

OPTICAL CROSS EXERCISES

1. Write the prescriptions in minus cylinder form:

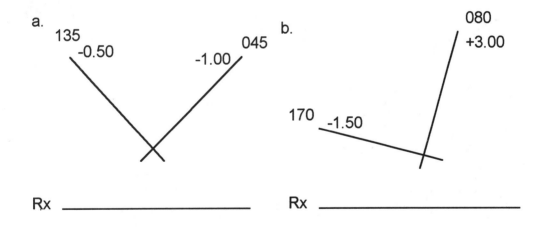

Rx _____

Rx _____

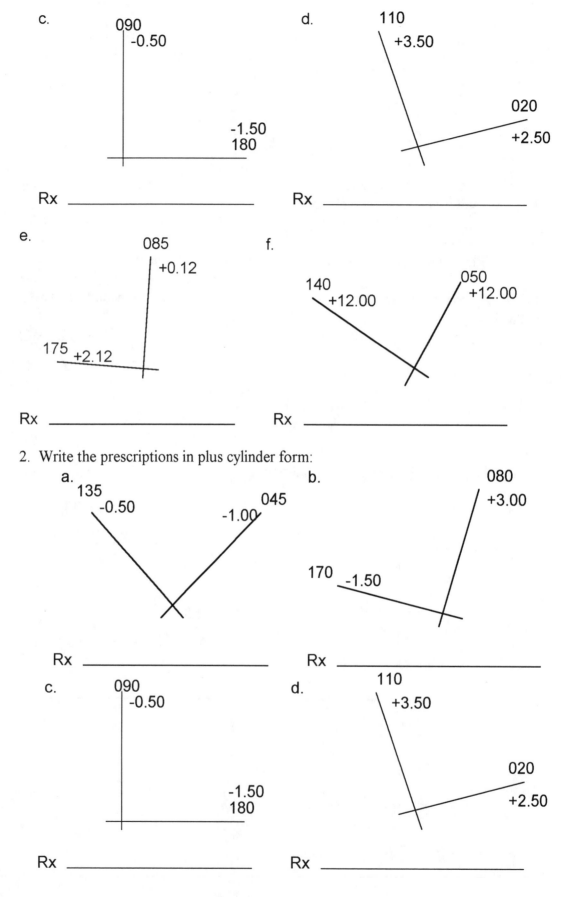

c.

090
-0.50

-1.50
180

Rx _____

d.

110
+3.50

020
+2.50

Rx _____

e.

085
+0.12

175 +2.12

Rx _____

f.

140
+12.00

050
+12.00

Rx _____

2. Write the prescriptions in plus cylinder form:

a.

135
-0.50

045
-1.00

Rx _____

b.

080
+3.00

170 -1.50

Rx _____

c.

090
-0.50

-1.50
180

Rx _____

d.

110
+3.50

020
+2.50

Rx _____

3. Write the prescriptions in cross cylinder form:

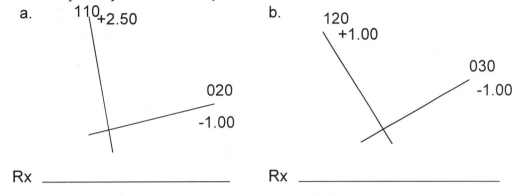

a.

110 +2.50

020
-1.00

b.

120
+1.00

030
-1.00

Rx _____

Rx _____

FLAT TRANSPOSITION

Some doctors write prescriptions in plus cylinder form, while others write prescriptions in minus cylinder form. The format is usually dictated by the equipment the doctor uses to refract. Some phoropters use plus cylinder lenses, and some phoropters use minus cylinder lenses.

Modern-day lenses are made in minus cylinder form, which means that the toric surface is the concave surface. Lenses made in plus cylinder form would have the toric surface on the convex side. The prescriber who writes the Rx in plus cylinder form does not intend that the lenses be made in that form unless there is a note on the Rx specifically requesting plus cylinder. If the prescription comes to us in plus cylinder form it may be necessary to rewrite it. We call this process flat transposition.

RULES FOR FLAT TRANSPOSITION:

1. New sphere: Algebraically add the spherical power and the cylinder.
2. New cylinder: Change the sign of the cylinder.
3. New axis: Change the axis by 90 degrees. If it is less than 90 degrees, add 90. If it is more than 90 degrees subtract 90.

EXAMPLE 1: Transpose the prescription +2.00 +1.00 x180 to minus cylinder form:
1. New sphere power:
Algebraically add the original spherical and cylindrical powers.
(+2.00) + (+1.00) = +3.00
2. New cylinder amount:
Change the sign of the original cylinder and keep the same cylinder amount.
+1.00 becomes −1.00
3. New axis power:
Add 90 degrees to the original axis if it is 90 degrees or lower. Subtract 90 degrees from the original axis if it is greater than 90 degrees.
180 − 90 = 090
Transposed Rx: +3.00 −1.00 x090.

Look back at the examples on pages 42 and 43. This transposed Rx and the original Rx resulted in the same lens, as shown on the optical cross.

EXAMPLE 2:   Transpose the Rx −3.50 +2.00 x020 to a minus cylinder.
1. New sphere: (−3.50) + (+2.00) = −1.50D
2. New cylinder: +2.00 becomes −2.00D
3. Axis: 020 + 90 = 110
The transposed Rx is −1.50 −2.00 x110.

Check the answer by placing both prescriptions on an optical cross. They are identical. We have not changed the Rx; we have only changed the way it was written.

FLAT TRANSPOSITION WORKSHEET

1. Transpose the following prescriptions into minus cylinder form.

a. −0.50 +1.50 x030   _____

b. +1.00 +3.00 x135   _____

c. −2.37 +1.50 x070   _____

2. Transpose the following prescriptions into plus cylinder form.

a. +2.00 −3.00 x060   _____

b. −1.00 −0.75 x140   _____

c. −1.62 −1.75 x065   _____

CROSS CYLINDER TRANSPOSITION

To determine the cross cylinder form of a prescription, either:
1. Put the prescription on an optical cross, and then remove it in cross cylinder form,
or
2. Flat transpose the prescription, and then cross connect the spheres and the axes.

EXAMPLE: What is the cross cylinder version of the Rx −1.00 +1.50 x110?

	Rx:	−1.00 +1.50 x110
Transposing gives:		+0.50 −1.50 x020

Cross connecting spheres: −1.00 +1.50 x110

+0.50 −1.50 x020

The Rx becomes   −1.00 x020 ☻ +0.50 x110

CROSS CYLINDER WORKSHEET

1. Rewrite the following prescriptions as cross cylinders:

   a. −1.00 +2.00 x090 ____________________

   b. +2.50 −3.62 x130 ____________________

   c. +1.00 −1.50 x096 ____________________

2. Rewrite the following cross cylinder prescriptions in minus cylinder form. (The optical cross may be helpful.)

   a. −1.00 x110 ⊕ +2.00 x020 ____________________

   b. +3.25 x080 ⊕ +1.00 x170 ____________________

   c. +10.50 x013 ⊕ +9.50 x103 ____________________

HAND NEUTRALIZATION

The term ***neutralization*** originated from the way the power of a lens used to be determined. When looking at the edge of a surface through a lens as the lens is moved, either the edge moves in the same direction as the lens movement, or the edge moves in the opposite direction from the lens movement.

A plus lens shows ***against movement***.

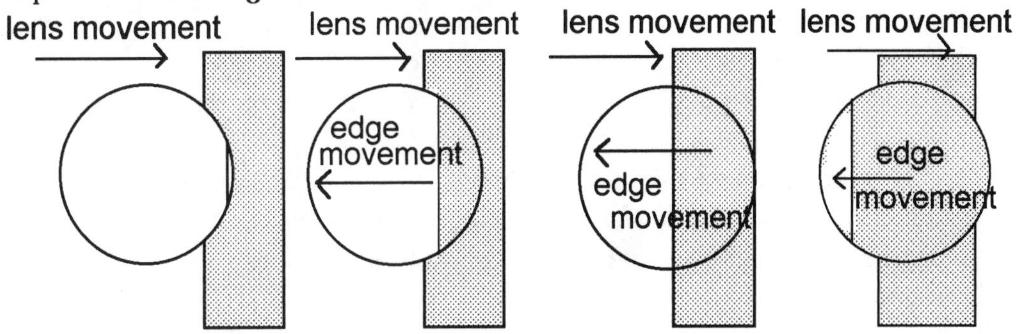

A minus lens shows ***with movement***.

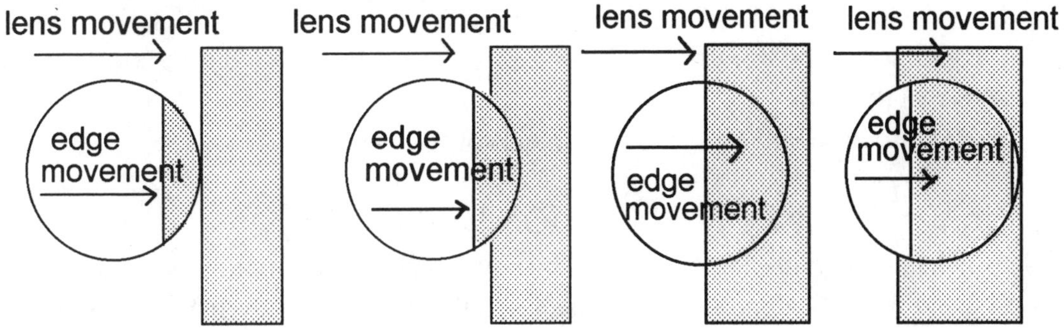

A plano lens shows no movement, or ***neutral movement***.

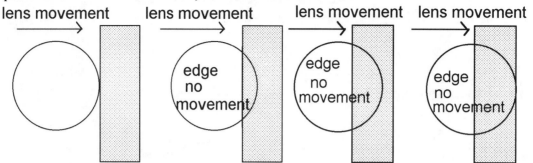

If we hold two lenses of opposite power together, they will *neutralize* each other's movement. If we can neutralize the movement of an unknown lens with a +5.00D lens, then the unknown lens must be a −5.00D lens.

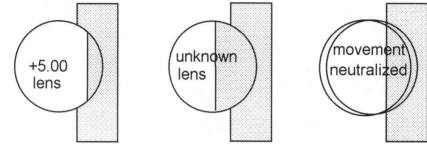

If we can neutralize the movement in only one direction with the +5.00D lens, but in the other direction we need a +6.00D lens, then the power in the first meridian is −5.00D, and in the second meridian the power is −6.00D.

EXAMPLE: In the horizontal meridian, a lens is hand-neutralized with a +1.00D lens, and in the vertical meridian the movement is neutralized with an *additional* +2.00D lens. What is the power of the lens?

1. Horizontal is the 180 degree meridian. Neutralization by a +1.00D lens means a power of −1.00D in this meridian in the unknown lens.
2. Vertical is the 90 degree meridian. Neutralization by adding +2.00D to the +1.00D already used means it took +3.00D to neutralize the movement. The power on the 90 degree meridian is −3.00D in the unknown lens.
3. The optical cross:

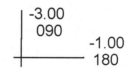

4. Removing the Rx from the optical cross gives an Rx of −1.00 −2.00 x180, or −3.00 +2.00 x090.

Note: The *additional* +2.00 lens gave the amount of the cylinder.

NEUTRALIZATION EXERCISES

1. A lens is hand neutralized and is found to show no horizontal motion when a −4.00D lens is used and no vertical motion when *just* a −2.00D lens is used. What is the power of the lens?

2. A lens is hand-neutralized and is found to show no horizontal motion when a +4.00D lens is used and no vertical motion when a +2.00D lens is *added* to the +4.00. What is the power of the lens?

3. A lens is hand neutralized and is found to show no horizontal motion when a +2.50D lens is used and no vertical motion when *just* a −1.00D lens is used. What is the power of the lens?

4. A lens is hand neutralized and is found to show no motion at about the 45 degree meridian when a −1.00D lens is used and no motion at about the 135 degree meridian when *an additional* −0.50D lens is included. What is the power of the lens?

5. Find a plus spherical lens, and a minus spherical lens, and try it for yourself!

PRESCRIPTION NOTATION

A. Sphere notation:
   1. Sign must be + or −.
   2. Value under +/−1.00D should have leading zero.
   3. Decimals are expressed to two places, and are in truncated eighths:
      0.12, 0.25, 0.37, 0.50, 0.62, 0.75, 0.87, 0.00
   4. A sphere power of 0.00 is written pl.
   5. D or DS may be used on non-compound Rx's; it is usually not
      entered for compound Rx's.

B. Cylinder notation:
   1. Sign must be + or −.
   2. Value under +/−1.00D should have leading zero.
   3. Decimals are expressed to two places, and are in truncated eighths:
      0.12, 0.25, 0.37, 0.50, 0.62, 0.75, 0.87, 0.00
   4. A cylinder power of 0.00 is not entered. Spherical Rx's use only the
      sphere power.
   5. D or DC is usually not entered.

C. Axis notation:
   1. Axis should be written with three digits: 001, 015, 155, etc.
   2. Axis is from 001 to 180. An axis of 000 is 180. Subtract 180 from
      any axis over 180.
   3. The degree sign is not written.

EXAMPLES: Corrected:

   1. +5.00 −0.00 x020 is a sphere with a zero cylinder power: +5.00, or +5.00DS.
   2. +5.00 − .5 x145 needs the cylinder rewritten as −0.50:   +5.00 −0.50 x145.
   3. +5.00 −0.50 x 225 needs the axis rewritten as 045:   +5.00 −0.50 x045.
   4. +5.00 −1.32 x050 needs the cylinder changed to −1.37:   +5.00 −1.37 x050.

5. 0.00 −3.00 x100 needs the sphere power rewritten pl: pl −3.00 x100

6. pl −3.00 x100° needs the degree sign dropped: pl −3.00 x100

7. 5.00 −0.50 x013 requires determining the sign of the sphere;
   it may *not* be assumed to be +. *Call the refractionist.*

8. pl −3.00 x 45 needs the axis rewritten as 045:   pl −3.00 x045.

Rx NOTATION EXERCISES

Decide what is wrong with the following (if anything) and correct it.

1. +8.5 −1.00 x15

2. 3.50 +1.50 x135

3. −.37 −1.50 x188

4. −1.37 +2.00 x115

5. +3.80 −.0.00 x132

6. +0.00 +0.62 x10°

7. +2.25 +2.12 x011

8. −3.00 0.75 x15

9. pl −0.87 x136

10. +4.37DS

11. −7.55

12. +.67 −.67 x10

13. −3.125 +3.125 x067

14. −1.11 − 0.00 x000

15. +0.50DS − 0.50DC x 210°

16. +20.50 −8.50 x045

CIRCLE OF LEAST CONFUSION

A spherical lens, having the same curvature in all meridians, brings the image of a distant point source to a point focus. A cylindrical lens is a lens that has one flat or plano side. A cylindrical lens brings the image of a distant point source to a line focus.

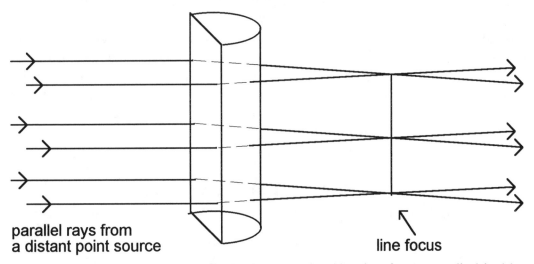

parallel rays from
a distant point source

line focus

A *compound lens*, or *spherocylinder lens*, can be thought of as two cylindrical lenses sandwiched together. When we showed the prescription in cross cylinder form, we were writing the prescription as two cylinders back-to-back. The compound lens brings the image of a distant point source to two line foci, one for each cylinder, instead of one point focus.

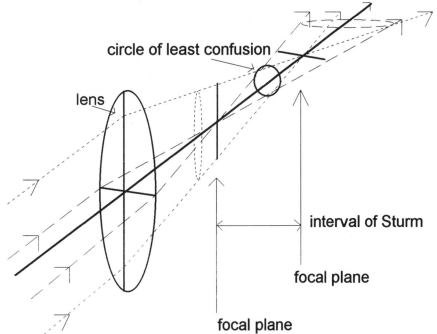

circle of least confusion

lens

interval of Sturm

focal plane

focal plane

The interval between the two focal lines in a compound lens is called the *interval of Sturm*. The length of the interval of Sturm is an indication of how long the *astigmatic interval* is. The interval of Sturm for a prescription is the difference between the focal lengths of the major meridian powers. The *toricity* of a surface is the difference between the two radii of curvature of the toric surface. The cylinder amount in the Rx notation is a way of judging the relative toricity of a lens, or comparing the astigmatic intervals of two lenses. The Rx −1.00 −4.00 x090 has a much longer astigmatic interval than does the Rx −1.00 −0.50 x090.

Between the two focal lines, light has a blurry and distorted focus. The plane where the focus has no distortion (but is still blurry) is the *circle of least confusion*.

The position of the circle of least confusion is found by taking the average of the powers in the two major meridians. This is the *spherical equivalent* of the Rx. The approximate distance of the circle of least confusion from the lens can be determined using the spherical equivalent for D in the focal power formula, D = 1/f. We use the spherical equivalent for initial contact lens selection, for base curve selection, and occasionally for approximating power or thickness.

SPHERICAL EQUIVALENT

To determine the spherical equivalent, add one-half of the amount of the cylinder to the sphere power:

$$D_{sph.eq.} = D_{sphere} + D_{cyl} / 2$$

EXAMPLE 1: What is the spherical equivalent of the Rx −2.00 −1.00 x090?
  1. 1/2 of the cylinder is (−1.00)/2 = −0.50.
  2. Add this amount to the sphere power: −2.00 + (−0.50) = −2.50.
  The spherical equivalent is −2.50D.
EXAMPLE 2: What is the spherical equivalent of the Rx +4.00 −3.00 x125?
  (+4.00) + (−3.00)/2 = (+4.00) + (−1.50) = **+2.50D.**
EXAMPLE 3: What is the spherical equivalent of the Rx −5.25D? Answer: −**5.25D.**

SPHERICAL EQUIVALENT EXERCISES
(Round to hundredths of a diopter.)

Determine the spherical equivalent for the following prescriptions:

1. −1.00 −0.50 x090 _____

2. pl −2.00 x170 _____

3. +2.00 −3.00 x025 _____

4. −1.25 +1.25 x160 _____

5. +1.00 +2.00 x060 _____

6. −0.50 +1.50 x030 _____

7. +1.00 +3.00 x135 _____

8. −2.37 +1.50 x070 _____

9. −1.00 −0.75 x140   _____

10. −1.62 −1.75 x065   _____

REFRACTIVE ERRORS

An *emmetropic eye* is an eye which, without accommodating, brings parallel incident light rays to a point focus on the retina. No correction is needed.

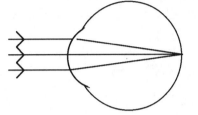

An *ametropic* eye is an eye which, without accommodating, does not bring parallel incident light rays to a point focus on the retina. Correction is needed in order to bring the distant focus to the retina.

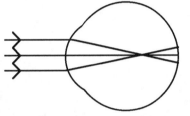

TYPES OF AMETROPIAS
1. HYPEROPIA or FARSIGHTEDNESS

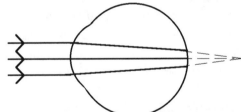

In hyperopia, parallel rays of light come to a focus behind the retina.

>   *Axial hyperopia*: The eye appears to be *too short.*
>   *Refractive hyperopia*: The refractive surfaces of the eye appear to be *too flat*, or the
>   eye has too little plus power.
>   Correction: Hyperopia requires a plus lens to add more power to the eye system,
>   increasing the convergence of the light rays and bringing parallel incident light
>   rays to a point focus on the retina.

Since light is absorbed by the retina the focus never actually falls behind the retina. In the case of all of the hyperopias discussed here, when we say the focus is behind the retina, we mean that the vergence is such that the focus would form behind the retina if the light continued to that point. In all cases of ametropia, when the focus is not on the retina, a blurred image forms on the retina. How blurred the image is depends on how far the focal plane is (or would be) from the retina.

2. MYOPIA or NEARSIGHTEDNESS

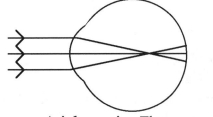

In myopia, parallel rays of light come to a focus in front of the retina.

Axial myopia: The eye appears to be *too long*.

Refractive myopia: The refractive surfaces of the eye appear to be *too steep*, or the eye has too much plus power.

Correction: Myopia requires a minus lens to reduce the convergence of the light rays, bringing parallel incident light rays to a point focus on the retina.

3. ASTIGMATISM

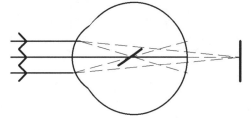

Astigmatism is a refractive error in which parallel rays of light do not come to a point focus on the retina. Instead, there are two line foci, corresponding to the maximum and minimum powers in the eye system.

Refractive: Almost all astigmatism is refractive. Astigmatism is usually the result of a toric cornea, or the crystalline lens being toric or tilted.

Regular astigmatism: The rays of light form two focal lines at 90 degrees from each other. This condition is corrected using compound or spherocylinder lenses.

Irregular astigmatism: A condition, usually caused by a damaged or irregular cornea, in which light rays form many focal lines, or form focal lines not at 90 degrees to each other. This condition cannot be corrected using spherocylindrical lenses, and usually requires the creation of a new optical surface. This new optical surface might be a contact lens or a corneal transplant.

REGULAR ASTIGMATISMS

1. SIMPLE ASTIGMATISM

A. *Simple Hyperopic Astigmatism* **(SHA)**

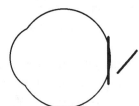

This is a condition where parallel rays of light come to two line foci, one falling on the retina and the other falling behind the retina.

An example of a prescription that corrects for SHA is: pl +2.00 x090, which can be transposed to +2.00 −2.00 x180.

B. *Simple Myopic Astigmatism* **(SMA)**

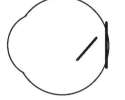

This is a condition where parallel rays of light come to two line foci, one falling on the retina and the other falling in front of the retina.

An example of a prescription that corrects for SMA is: pl −2.00 x090, which can be transposed to −2.00 +2.00 x180.

2. COMPOUND ASTIGMATISM

A. *Compound Hyperopic Astigmatism* **(CHA)**

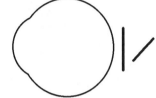

This is a condition where parallel rays of light come to two line foci, both of which fall behind the retina.

An example of a prescription that corrects for CHA is: +1.00 +2.00 x090, which can be transposed to +3.00 −2.00 x180.

B. *Compound Myopic Astigmatism* **(CMA)**

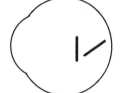

This is a condition where parallel rays of light come to two line foci, both of which fall in front of the retina.

An example of a prescription that corrects for CMA is: −1.00 −2.00 x090, which can be transposed to −3.00 +2.00 x180.

3. MIXED ASTIGMATISM (MA)

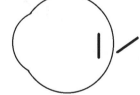

This is a condition where parallel rays of light come to two line foci, one falling in front of the retina and the other falling behind the retina.

An example of a prescription that corrects for MA is +1.00 −1.50 x090, which can be transposed to −0.50 +1.50 x180.

REFRACTIVE ERRORS EXERCISES

Determine the refractive error illustrated by the following diagrams.

H   Hyperopia
M   Myopia
SHA   Simple Hyperopic Astigmatism
SMA   Simple Myopic Astigmatism
CHA   Compound Hyperopic Astigmatism
CMA   Compound Myopic Astigmatism
MA   Mixed Astigmatism

1.

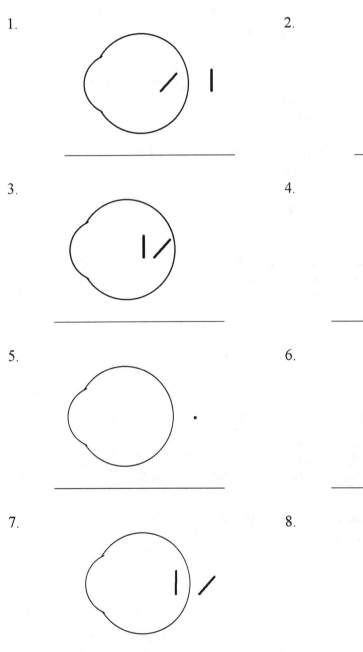

2.

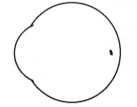

_____

3.

4.

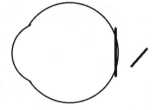

_____

5.

6.

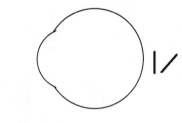

_____

7.

8.

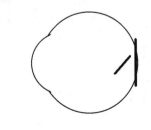

_____

EVALUATING THE ASTIGMATISM

To determine the wearer's visual abnormality, flat transpose the prescription and then consider the powers in the major meridians.

POWERS IN MAJOR MERIDIANS	REFRACTIVE ERROR	
PL +	(SHA)	Simple Hyperopic Astigmatism
PL –	(SMA)	Simple Myopic Astigmatism
+ + (unequal power)	(CHA)	Compound Hyperopic Astigmatism
– – (unequal power)	(CMA)	Compound Myopic Astigmatism
+ –	(MA)	Mixed Astigmatism

EXAMPLE: +3.00 –1.00 x135: flat transposition gives +2.00 +1.00 x045. The two major powers are both +. Therefore, the prescription corrects for CHA.

EVALUATING THE ASTIGMATISM EXERCISES

Determine the nature of the refractive error for the following prescriptions:

1. –1.00 –0.50 x090   _____CMA_____

2. pl –2.00 x170   _____SMA_____

3. +2.00 –3.00 x025   _____MA_____

4. –1.25 +1.25 x160   _____

5. +1.00 +2.00 x060   _____

6. –0.50 +1.50 x030   _____

7. +1.00 +3.00 x135   _____

8. –2.37 +1.50 x070   _____

9. +2.00 –0.75 x140   _____

10. +1.62 –1.62 x065   _____

WITH AND AGAINST THE RULE ASTIGMATISM

With the rule astigmatism

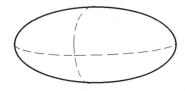

Astigmatism is said to be with the rule if the steepest meridian of the cornea or the crystalline lens is near the vertical meridian. In this case, the correction requires using a plus cylinder with axis near 90 degrees, or a minus cylinder with axis near 180 degrees.

Against the rule astigmatism

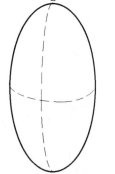

Astigmatism is said to be against the rule if the steepest meridian of the cornea or the crystalline lens is near the horizontal meridian. In this case, the correction requires using a plus cylinder with axis near 180 degrees, or a minus cylinder with axis near 90 degrees.

Note: The term "with the rule" comes from the fact that the majority of astigmatic people have the steepest meridian on the vertical direction of the cornea.

Oblique astigmatism

Astigmatism is said to be oblique if it is more than 30° away from the horizontal or the vertical meridians. An example of this would be the Rx −2.00 +1.00 x055, or +1.50 −0.50 x132.

To determine whether an Rx corrects for with the rule or against the rule astigmatism, look at the written prescription and the sign and axis of the cylinder.

WR – with the rule astigmatism:
 minus cylinder form, axis within 30 degrees of the 180 meridian; or plus cylinder form, axis within 30 degrees of the 90 meridian.

AR – against the rule astigmatism:
 minus cylinder form, axis within 30 degrees of the 90 meridian; or plus cylinder form, axis within 30 degrees of the 180 meridian.

O – oblique astigmatism:
 cylinder axis from 31 to 59 degrees, or cylinder axis from 121 to 149 degrees.

You may find it easier to remember the following peacock's tail, which requires the Rx to be in *minus cylinder form*:

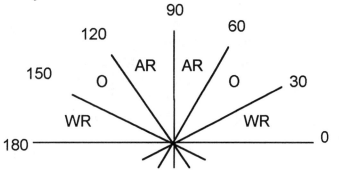

EXAMPLES:
1. +3.00 −1.00 x050   Oblique
2. +3.00 −1.00 x155   With the rule
3. +3.00 +1.00 x003   Against the rule
4. +3.00 +1.00 x130   Oblique

WITH AND AGAINST THE RULE ASTIGMATISM EXERCISES

Determine whether the following prescriptions correct for with the rule, against the rule, or oblique astigmatism.

1. −1.00 −1.00 x180   _____

2. −0.50 −2.00 x050   _____

3. −0.50 + 2.00 x080   _____

4. +0.75 −1.50 x110   _____

5. +2.00 + 0.50 x090   _____

6. −1.25 −0.75 x130   _____

7. +1.00 +3.00 x115   _____

8. −2.37 +1.50 x070   _____

9. −1.00 +0.75 x140   _____

10. −1.62 −1.75 x065   _____

POWER IN OBLIQUE MERIDIANS

We learned that a cylinder exerts all of its power 90 degrees from its axis, and no power along its axis. The approximate power of a lens in any particular meridian varies between the powers in the two major meridians.

In optics, we often need to know the approximate power of a lens in a meridian other than its axis, such as when determining how much prism has been created when the pupillary distance is incorrect, or how much to move the lens in order to include prescribed prism, or in computing vertical imbalance, or computing image jump. All of these subjects will be covered in this book.

To find the approximate power of a lens in any meridian on the lens, use the *oblique meridian formula*:

$$D_T = D_S + D_C (\sin \alpha)^2$$

where D_T is the total power in the desired meridian,
D_S is the power of the sphere in the Rx,
D_C is the power of the cylinder in the Rx,
α is the angle between the axis in the Rx and the meridian we want.

As an alternative to using the formula, memorize:

> A cylinder exerts 100% of its power 90 degrees from its axis.
> A cylinder exerts   75% of its power 60 degrees from its axis.
> A cylinder exerts   50% of its power 45 degrees from its axis.
> A cylinder exerts   25% of its power 30 degrees from its axis.
> A cylinder exerts 0% of its power on axis.

Look at the second diagram on page 53. The powers of the two major meridians are the two distances at which light is brought to a line focus. In between these two distances a piece of film would show a blurred and distorted image, not a sharp line image. When using the focimeter or lensometer, there are two powers that give clearly focused lines: the powers between result in blurred images. Although we routinely refer to the 'power' on a meridian other than the axis of the Rx, keep in mind that the lens does not *actually* have that power at that meridian.

EXAMPLE 1: What is the approximate total power along the vertical (90th) meridian for the Rx −1.00 −2.00 x060?

D_T = ?	$D_T = D_S + D_C(\sin \alpha)^2$
D_S = −1.00D	$D_T = -1.00 + -2.00\,(\sin 30)^2$
D_C = −2.00D	$D_T = -1.00 + (-2.00 \times 0.25)$
α = 90 −60 = 30	$D_T = -1.00 + (-0.50)$
	$\mathbf{D_T = -1.50D}$

Alternatively the desired meridian is 30 degrees from the axis of the Rx. The cylinder exerts 25% of its power 30 degrees away. 25% of −2.00D is −0.50. Adding −0.50 to the sphere power of −1.00 gives −1.50D.

EXAMPLE 2: What is the approximate total power on the horizontal meridian for the Rx +2.25 −1.00 x060?

180 − 60 = 120; or 60 to 0 is 60. Using either 60 or 120 for the angle α will give the correct result.

$$\mathbf{D_T} = (+2.25) + (-1.00)(\sin 60)^2 = (+2.25) + (-1.00)(0.75)$$
$$= (+2.25) + (-0.75) = \mathbf{+1.50D}$$

Or, 75% of the cylinder is in effect 60 degrees from the axis; 75% of −1.00 is −0.75; +2.25 − 0.75 is +1.50D.

EXAMPLE 3: What is the approximate total power of a −4.50 −2.50 x125 lens on the horizontal meridian?

180 − 125 = 55 degrees

$$\mathbf{D_T} = (-4.50) + (-2.50)(\sin 55)^2 = (-4.50) + (-2.50)(0.67)$$
$$= (-4.50) + (-1.68) = \mathbf{-6.18D}$$

The shortcut is not usable in this case, but do check what the answer should be close to by noticing that 55 degrees is close to 60 degrees; so just under 75% of the cylinder is in effect, which comes to −1.87DC. The total at 60 degrees away would be −6.37D. Our answer is just a little less than that, which is what we would expect.

OBLIQUE MERIDIAN FORMULA EXERCISE
(Round to hundredths of a diopter.)

1. What is the approximate total power in the horizontal meridian for the Rx
    −2.00 +3.00 x045?

2. What is the approximate total power in the vertical meridian for the Rx
    −4.00 −2.00 x180?

3. What is the approximate total power in the 140 degree meridian for the Rx
    +3.00 −1.00 x080?

4. How much *cylinder power* is in effect along the 35 degree meridian in the Rx
    −2.50 +4.00 x065?

5. What is the approximate total power on the 180 meridian of the Rx
    +6.00 −1.50 x112?

6. What is the approximate total power on the 90th meridian for the Rx
    −10.25 +3.50 x 62?

VERTEX DISTANCE AND EFFECTIVE POWER

In any optical system, a lens effectively gains in plus power as it moves away from the rest of the system. This effective gain in plus power is the basis for focusable camera lenses. A plus lens placed in front of an eye becomes part of an optical system. The plus lens will *effectively* get stronger as it moves away from the eye, and the plus lens will *effectively* get weaker as it moves toward the eye. The **effective power** of the lens changes based on its distance from the eye, even though the lens itself does not change.

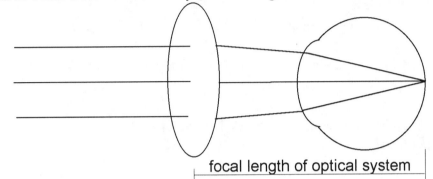

focal length of optical system

This plus lens is the correct power and distance away from the eye to focus parallel incident light rays on the retina. The focal length of the optical system consisting of lens plus eye is exactly the distance from the lens to the retina.

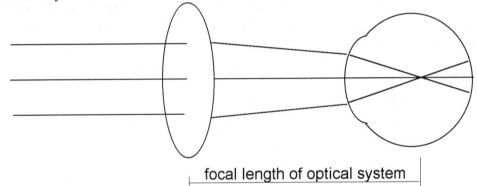

focal length of optical system

The same lens moved away from the eye results in the optical system having too short a focal length. The lens has *effectively* gained plus power. The effective power of the lens with respect to the optical system comprised of lens plus eye is now too strong. *As a lens moves away from the eye, it gains plus power or loses minus power.*

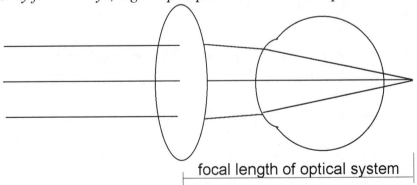

focal length of optical system

The same lens moved toward the eye results in the optical system having too long a focal length. The lens has *effectively* lost plus power. The effective power of the lens with respect to the optical system comprised of lens and eye is now too weak. *As a lens moves toward the eye, it loses plus power or gains minus power.*

Likewise, the effective power of a minus lens will decrease as it is moved away from the eye. The minus lens is gaining plus, thus decreasing its effective power. As the minus lens moves toward the eye it loses plus power, effectively making it a stronger minus lens.

The vertex distance is an indication of how far the ocular (or back) side of the lens is from the corneal apex. This is measured with a distometer.

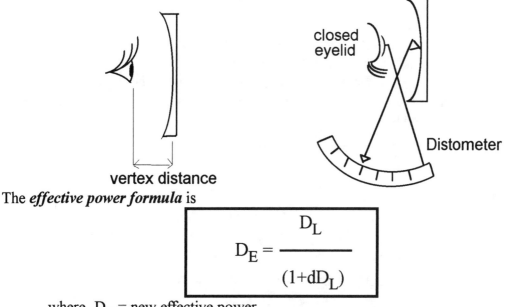

vertex distance

The *effective power formula* is

$$D_E = \frac{D_L}{(1+dD_L)}$$

where D_E = new effective power,

D_L = original lens power,

d = change in vertex distance in meters.

If the lens is moved toward the eye, d is positive. If the lens is moved away from the eye, d is negative. (We try to get people to choose glasses that will sit close to the eye: a good way to remember the sign of d is that closer is good, i.e., positive.)

[As an alternative method, disregard the signs of both d and D_L in the denominator: if the result is to be a stronger power, use a denominator of $(1 - dD_L)$, and if the result is to be weaker power, use a denominator of $(1+dD_L.)$]

EXAMPLE 1: The Rx reads OD −6.00D, refracted VD 10mm. The glasses fit at 13mm. If no adjustment is made to the prescription, what is the effective power of the −6.00D lens?

d = −3mm = −0.003meters (negative because the lens is moving away.)

$$D_E = \frac{D_L}{1 + dD_L} = \frac{-6.00}{1+(-0.003)\,(-6.00)} = \frac{-6.00}{1.018}$$

$D_E = -5.89D$

[Alternatively, disregard all signs in the denominator. Since the lens is a minus lens and is moving away from the eye, it will gain plus power or lose minus power. Therefore the effective power will be less than -6.00, so the denominator is $1+dD_L = 1+(0.003)(6.00) = 1.018$.]

There is an approximation formula that many people use: the *change in power* is equal to $dD^2/1000$, where d *is measured in mm*. In the above example, this gives $(3)(6.00)^2/1000 = 0.108 = 0.11D$ change. Since the lens is a minus lens moving away from the wearer's eye, the lens gains plus power or loses minus power, and the effective power is approximately $-6.00 + 0.11 = -5.89$.

EXAMPLE 2: The Rx reads OD $+15.00D$, refracted VD 14mm. The wearer is to be fitted with contact lenses, vertex distance $= 0$mm. If the fitter starts with a $+15.00$ contact lens, what is the effective power that the wearer will experience?

$d = +14$mm $= +0.014$meters (positive because the lens is moving toward the eye).

$$D_E = \frac{D_L}{1 + dD_L} = \frac{+15.00}{1+(+0.014)\,(+15.00)} = \frac{+15.00}{1.21}$$

$$\mathbf{D_E = +12.40D}$$

[Alternatively, disregard all signs in the denominator. Since the lens is a plus lens and is moving toward the eye, it will lose plus power. Therefore, the effective power will be less than $+15.00$, so the denominator is $1+dD_L = 1+(0.014)(15.00) = 1.21$.]

In the second example, the approximation formula for the change in power = $dD^2/1000 = (14)(15)^2/1000 = 3.15D$ change in power. The lens is a plus lens moving toward the eye; thus, it loses in plus power. The effective power is $+15.00 - 3.15 = +11.85D$. This is not a very good approximation of the actual answer. The approximation formula is good only for small vertex distance changes or low lens powers.

When computing effective power for a toric lens, compute the powers in the major meridians separately, and then convert back to Rx notation. The optical cross is a good tool to use for this.

EXAMPLE 3: The Rx reads OD balance, OS $-9.00 -2.50$ x154, refracted at 10mm. The glasses fit at 8mm. If no adjustment is made to the left eye prescription, what effective power will the wearer experience?

The powers in the major meridians are $-9.00D$ and $-11.50D$. The lens is moving 2mm toward the eye, so $d = +2$mm $= +0.002$m.

The effective power on the 154 meridian is:

$$D_E = \frac{D_L}{1 + dD_L} = \frac{-9.00}{1+(+0.002)\,(-9.00)} = \frac{-9.00}{0.982}$$

D_E on the 154 meridian $= -9.16D$

The effective power on the 064 meridian is:

$$D_E = \frac{D_L}{1 + dD_L} = \frac{-11.50}{1+(+0.002)\,(-11.50)} = \frac{-11.50}{0.977}$$

$$D_E \text{ on the 064 meridian} = -11.77D$$

Using the optical cross to see what is happening:
-9.00 -2.50 x 154

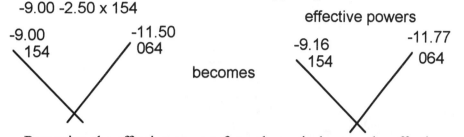

Removing the effective powers from the optical cross, the effective prescription is **−9.16 −2.61 x154**. Notice that if you performed the calculations on the −2.50 cylinder instead of the actual power in the 064 meridian, the effective cylinder amount would appear to be −2.51 instead of −2.61. This answer would underestimate the effect of moving the lens without compensating for the power change.

When determining the *actual effective power*, do not change to one-eighth diopter steps. Round to two decimal places. We are *not* going to order or make this lens.

EFFECTIVE POWER EXERCISE
(Round to hundredths of a diopter.)

1. The Rx is   OD −5.00D   refracted at 10mm VD
              OS −6.50D

   What are the effective powers if this person is fitted with contact lenses of these powers? (New vertex distance is 0mm.)

2. The Rx is   OD +5.00 +2.00 x090   refracted at 8mm
              OS +6.00 +2.50 x145

   What is the effective power of the lenses if the glasses made of this prescription are worn with a vertex distance of 14mm?

   Note: Powers in the major meridians in the OD are +5.00D and +7.00D. Use the formula to find the effective power in each of these meridians, then convert back to the Rx notation. You may wish to use the optical cross. What are the major meridian powers in the OS?

COMPENSATED POWER

For high-power prescriptions that will be worn at a vertex distance other than the refracted distance, we need to determine what power lens to order so that the wearer will be looking through the power intended by the prescriber. This is the *compensated* or *recomputed* power.

The compensated power formula is

$$D_C = \frac{D_L}{(1 - dD_L)}$$

where D_C = compensated power (what will be ordered),
D_L = original lens power,
d = change in vertex distance in meters.

If the lens is moved toward the eye, d is positive. If the lens is moved away from the eye, d is negative.

Or, disregard the signs of d and D_L in the denominator: if the result is to be a stronger power use $(1-dD_L)$, and if the result is to be a weaker power use $(1+dD_L)$.

EXAMPLE 1: The Rx reads OD −6.00D, refracted VD 10mm.
The glasses fit at 13mm. What power lens should be ordered so that the wearer will be looking through the power intended by the refractionist?

$$D_C = \frac{D_L}{1 - dD_L} = \frac{-6.00}{1 - (-0.003)(-6.00)} = \frac{-6.00}{0.982}$$

$$D_C = -6.11D \text{ (order it } -6.12D)$$

[Alternatively, disregard all signs in the denominator. Since the lens is a minus lens and is moving away from the eye, it will gain plus power or lose minus power. Therefore it would be ordered as more than −6.00, and the denominator is $1-dD_L = 1-(0.003)(6.00) = 0.982$.]

Or, use the approximation formula, change = $dD^2/1000$, where d is in mm. The result is $(3)(6.00)^2/1000 = 0.108$. Since the lens is negative and is moving away from the eye, a stronger lens would be ordered, so the result is −6.00 −0.11 = −6.11D. Order −6.12D.

EXAMPLE 2: The Rx reads OD balance, OD −9.00 −2.50 x154, refracted at 10mm. The glasses fit at 8mm. What power lens should be ordered so that the wearer will be looking through the power intended by the refractionist?

The powers in the major meridians are −9.00D and −11.50D. The lens is moving 2mm toward the eye, so d = +2mm = +0.002m.

The compensated power on the 154 meridian is:

$$D_C = \frac{D_L}{1 - dD_L} = \frac{-9.00}{1-(+0.002)\,(-9.00)} = \frac{-9.00}{1.018}$$

D_C on the 154 meridian = $-8.84D$

The compensated power on the 064 meridian is:

$$D_C = \frac{D_L}{1 - dD_L} = \frac{-11.50}{1-(+0.002)\,(-11.50)} = \frac{-11.50}{1.023}$$

D_C on the 064 meridian = $-11.24D$

Using the optical cross to see what is happening:

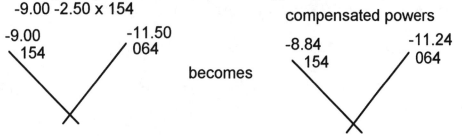

Removing the compensated powers from the optical cross, the prescription becomes -8.84 -2.40 x154, which changes to **-8.87 -2.37 x154**. Notice that if you performed the calculations on the -2.50 cylinder instead of the actual power in the 064 meridian, the effective cylinder amount would appear to be -2.49 instead of -2.40, and would round to -2.50 cylinder. This answer would result in ordering the prescription with too much cylinder power.

WHAT YOU REALLY NEED TO KNOW
COMPENSATED POWER: order:

lens moves:	away from eye	toward eye
plus lens	weaker	stronger
minus lens	stronger	weaker

Note: The compensated power is changed to eighths of a diopter, while the effective power is not. The effective power is what the wearer is *actually seeing*. The compensated power w*ill be made in the laboratory*. We change to eighths when we are going to actually order or make the lens. If the answer is halfway between two 1/8D increments, change to the next smaller 1/8D.

Note: Adjusting the prescription for vertex distance changes is the only time that an optician may order a lens power that is different from the prescription written by the refractionist. It is good policy to call the refractionist and request permission to order the compensated power. At this time, indicate what the new power will be, so that it may be recorded in the wearer's records. When fitting contact lenses it is not necessary to request permission from the refractionist, since calculating compensating power is part of the contact lens fitting procedure.

COMPENSATED POWER EXERCISES
(Change to eighths of a diopter.)

1. The Rx is   OD −5.00D   refracted at 10mm VD
                 OS −6.50D

   If the Rx was to be dispensed as contact lenses what powers contact lenses would you *start* the fitting with? (Contact lenses have a vertex distance of 0.)

2. The Rx is   OD +5.00 +2.00 x090   refracted at 8mm
                    OS +6.00 +2.50 x145

   What lens powers would be ordered for glasses that are to be worn with a vertex distance of 14mm?

EFFECTIVE AND COMPENSATED POWER EXERCISES

3. A myope receives a prescription of   OD −6.50 −2.00 x090
                                          OS −8.25 −0.25 x090.
                                   refracted VD 10mm.

   The glasses chosen are at 13mm vertex distance.

   a. What effective power would the wearer be looking through if the above prescription were ordered as is?

   b. What prescription could be ordered to compensate for the vertex distance?

   c. The person decided to try contact lenses. What would be the *starting point* for the lens power? (Change the answers to the nearest 0.25D. Adjust the result to what is available in this power range in the C.L. of choice.)

   d. The daughter wants her mother to have "nice big stylish frames" that fit at 17mm vertex distance. What power would be ordered for these glasses?

SECTION IV: PRISMS

PRISM DEFINITIONS

A prism is formed by any two flat surfaces inclined at an angle to one another.

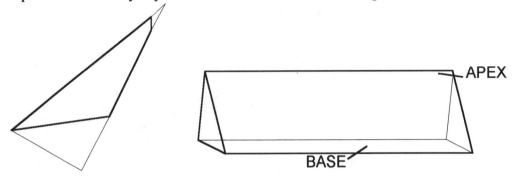

We usually think of a prism as a transparent wedge.

A prism has a base and an apex. We call the angle made at the apex the *apical angle*, or the *apex angle*, or the *refracting angle*, or the *prism angle*. Any of these terms may be used.

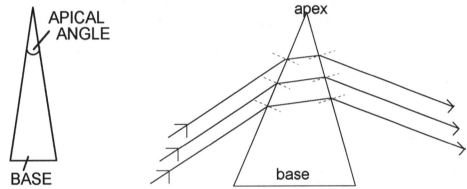

A prism has no focal power. A prism deviates the light passing through it, but does not change its vergence. Light passing through a prism undergoes refraction at both surfaces and exits refracted or *deviated* toward the base.

When a beam of light passes through a prism, the three D's occur: *Dispersion, Displacement*, and *Deviation*.

DISPERSION OF LIGHT BY A PRISM

Dispersion is defined as the breaking up of white light into its component or *spectral* colors. Different wavelengths of white light travel at the same speed in air, but travel at different speeds in more dense materials.

Red light travels faster than violet light in transparent materials other than air. When a ray of light enters a prism, each of its component colors is refracted a different amount at each of the prism's surfaces. The blue end of the spectrum is refracted more than the red end because the blue waves are slowed more than the red waves. Use the name **ROY G. BIV** to help remember the colors from longest wavelength and least refraction to shortest wavelength and most refraction.

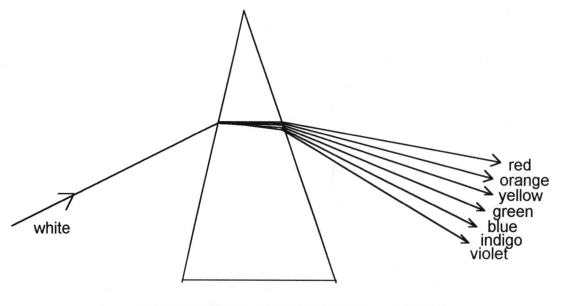

OBJECT DISPLACEMENT BY A PRISM

An object viewed through a prism appears to be in a different place than if viewed without the prism. The object always appears to be *displaced* toward the apex of the prism.

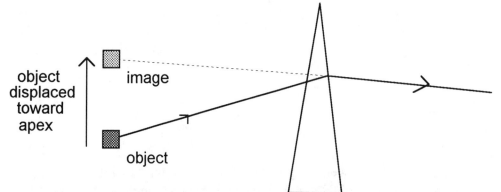

Because the image seen through the prism is displaced toward the apex, the eye will turn toward the apex in order to view the image. An eye can be made to turn up, down, in or out by placing prism in front of it. A *relieving* or *therapeutic* prism is placed in front of an eye with a weak or paralyzed muscle to displace the image in the same direction that the eye turns. In this case, the base of the prism is placed over the weak muscle, sending the image in the same direction that the eye is turning. *Adverse prism* or *exercising prism* is placed with the apex over the weak muscle to make it work harder. This technique may be used during eye exercises designed to strengthen the weak muscle.

The human eye is sensitive to small amounts of prism. Unwanted or unintentional prism will result in discomfort for the wearer.

PRISM POWER

There are four different prism power units in use:

Apical or *refracting angle* (discussed on page 71)
Deviating angle
Centrad
Prism diopter (the unit used by the optical industry and defined in ANSI Z80.1-1995)

DEVIATING ANGLE

The *deviating angle* is similar to the angle of deviation used when we originally discussed refraction in Section III. The deviating angle, δ, is the angle formed by the emerging ray with the path that the ray would have taken had the prism not been present.

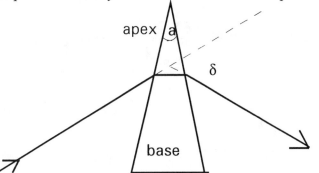

The deviating angle is related to the apical angle, a, by the approximation formula

$$\delta = a\,(n - 1)$$

This formula is an approximation for small a and δ, so it is not useful for strong prisms. The formula can be rewritten as

$$a = \delta\,/\,(n - 1)$$

EXAMPLE 1: If a prism made of crown glass (n=1.523) has an apical angle of 5 degrees, what is its angle of deviation?

$$\delta = 5\,(1.523 - 1) = 5 \times 0.523 = 2.6 \text{ degrees}$$

EXAMPLE 2: If a crown glass prism is needed that will change the path of incoming light rays by 12 degrees, what apical angle will the prism be manufactured with?

$$a = 12\,/\,(1.523 - 1) = 12\,/\,0.523 = 22.9 \text{ degrees}$$

ANGLE OF DEVIATION EXERCISES
(Round angles to the nearest one-tenth.)

1. What angle of deviation would a prism made of flint glass (n = 1.70) have if it were made with an apical angle of 17 degrees?

2. A prism deviates light by 18 degrees, and is made out of CR39 (n = 1.498). What is the apical angle of the prism?

3. A prism with a 10 degree apical angle deviates incident light by 6 degrees. What is the index of refraction of the material that the prism is made of?

CENTRAD

The **_centrad_** measures the amount that an image is displaced by a prism. When we look at an object and then move a prism in front of our eyes, the image of the object "jumps" or moves a certain amount. How far the image appears to move depends on how far away the object is from the prism and how strong the prism is.

When the prism displaces the image, the distance that the image moves can be traced out on a circle that has, as its radius, the distance the object is from the prism. One measurement used for angles by scientists and mathematicians is the radian; a centrad is one one-hundredth of a radian. If radians are used to measure the angle of deviation, δ, then a one centrad deviation would be equivalent to the image moving one one-hundredth of a meter _on the circumference of a circle_ if the object is one meter away from the prism.

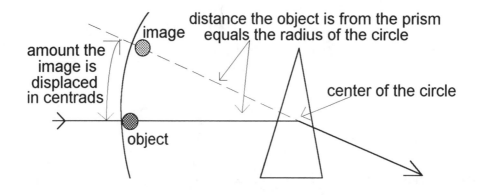

This is the most accurate measurement of displacement and is used for very strong prisms. It is denoted by an inverted triangle ∇.

PRISM DIOPTER

The prism diopter is denoted by the Greek letter delta Δ. This unit of prism measurement was proposed by C.F. Prentice in 1888 and is the unit which is used in the ophthalmic laboratory. It is actually an approximation of the centrad. It is close enough to the centrad for our purposes, as long as we are dealing with prisms that have a deviation of less than about 10 degrees or an apical angle of less than about 15 degrees.

A prism diopter produces a displacement of 1 unit (along a straight line) at a distance of 100 units. In more common usage, a prism diopter produces an image displacement of 1 centimeter at an object distance of 1 meter. The difference between the prism diopter and the centrad is that the centrad measures the distance along the arc of a circle instead of along a straight line.

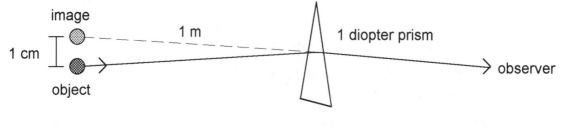

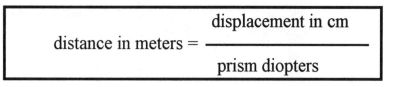

$$\text{PRISM DIOPTER} = \frac{\text{DISPLACEMENT IN CENTIMETERS}}{\text{DISTANCE IN METERS}}$$

EXAMPLE: What is the power of a prism that produces a 2cm displacement when the object is 3m away?

$$P^\Delta = \text{displacement (cm)/distance (m)} = 2/3 = 0.67^\Delta$$

The formula may be rewritten to find either distance of object or displacement of image:

$$\boxed{\text{Displacement in cm} = \text{prism diopters} \times \text{distance in meters}}$$

$$\text{distance in meters} = \frac{\text{displacement in cm}}{\text{prism diopters}}$$

EXAMPLE: How much and in what direction will an object be displaced when viewed through a 3^Δ prism held base down 2 meters from the object?

Displacement in cm = prism diopters × distance in meters

$$= 3 \times 2 = 6cm$$

Since the prism is being held base down and the object is displaced toward the apex, the image will appear to be 6cm higher than the position of the object.

Note: The distance that the image is displaced from the object is a straight line. This distance is very close to equal to the distance on the arc of the circle discussed for the centrad. For small prisms, less than 10^Δ, or for small apical angles, less than $15°$, the prism diopter is an accurate measurement. For strong prisms, the centrad is more accurate than the prism diopter. For these strong prisms the prism diopter overestimates the power of the prism.

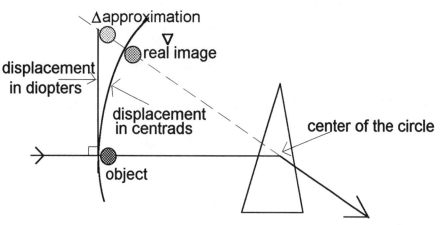

PRISM DIOPTER DISPLACEMENT EXERCISES

1. What power prism would displace an object to the left by 2 cm when viewed through a prism that is 2m away from the object?

2. How much displacement would a 2 diopter prism held base up cause in an object 4m from the prism?

3. A 2 diopter prism makes an object viewed through it appear to be displaced 3cm lower than it is. How far is the object from the prism, and what is its base direction?

RELATIONSHIP BETWEEN PRISM DEFINITIONS

The prism diopter is related to the angle of deviation and the apical angle. The relationship for the deviating angle and prism diopter is

$$P = 100 \tan \delta$$

where P = power in prism diopters,
       δ = angle of deviation.

Substituting $\delta = a (n - 1)$ into this equation we also have the approximation

$$P = 100 \tan [a(n-1)]$$

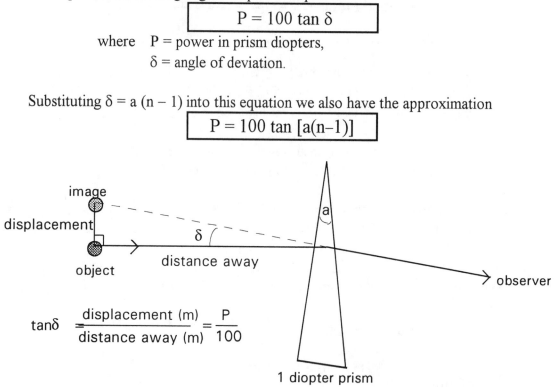

$$\tan\delta = \frac{\text{displacement (m)}}{\text{distance away (m)}} = \frac{P}{100}$$

1 diopter prism

EXAMPLE 1: What is the power in prism diopters of a crown glass (n = 1.523) prism having an apical angle of 5°?

    $P = 100 \tan [a(n-1)] = 100 \tan [5(1.523-1)] = 100 \tan [2.615] = 4.6^\Delta$

EXAMPLE 2: What apical angle would a prism need to have if it is made of polycarbonate (n = 1.586) and is to have a power of 6^Δ?

    a. P = 100 tan δ b. $\delta = a(n-1)$
         tan δ = 6/100   3.4 = a(1.586-1)
         $\delta = 3.4°$ a = 3.4/0.586 = 5.8°

MORE PRISM DIOPTER EXERCISES
(Round angles and prism diopters to one-tenth.)

1. If a prism is to have a power of 3.5$^\Delta$, what deviating angle will it have?

2. If a prism is to be made out of CR39 (n = 1.498) and have a power of 3.5$^\Delta$, what apical angle should it have?

3. If a prism has an apical angle of 8° and a power of 8.4$^\Delta$, what is the index of refraction of the material it is made from?

THE LENS AS A PRISM

Any lens can be caricatured as a set of prisms. Plus lenses act like two prisms with their bases together. Minus lenses act like two prisms with their apices together.

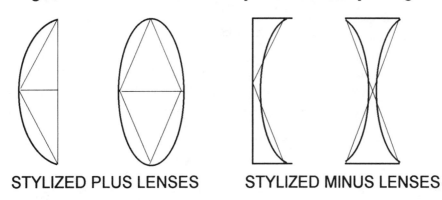

STYLIZED PLUS LENSES   STYLIZED MINUS LENSES

The power of any lens may be considered to be the result of the prismatic effect created by the incline of the surfaces with respect to each other at any particular point on the lens. We can look at the lens as if it were a series of different power prisms stacked on top of one another. Take a look at the "stacked prisms" in the diagrams:

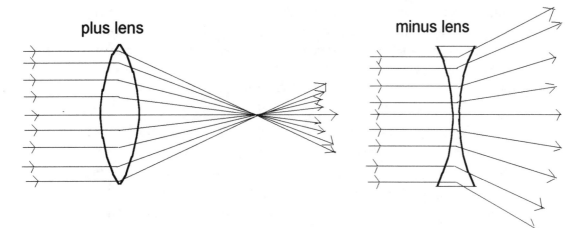

plus lens   minus lens

At the center of the lens the sides are parallel, there is no prism power, and the ray (or axis) is not bent or deviated. A ray traveling through the lens at any other point on the lens is bent or deviated based on the incline of the sides at that point. The further from the center of the lens, the more the sides are inclined with respect to each other, and the more the ray is deviated.

IMAGE MOVEMENT

Objects viewed through the center of a lens will not be displaced, since there is no prism present at the center of the lens. Objects viewed through points other than the center will be displaced toward the apex of the prism. In a plus lens, the object is displaced away from the optical center. In a minus lens, the object is displaced toward the optical center.

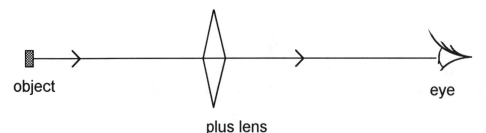

As a plus lens is moved down, an object viewed through the lens will be displaced upwards toward the apex of the prism created by the lens. This is called *against movement* or *against motion*. The speed of the against movement is greater for a high power plus lens than for a low power plus lens.

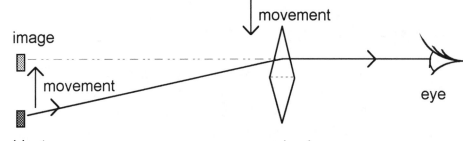

As a minus lens is moved down, an object viewed through the lens will be displaced down toward the apex of the prism created by the lens. This is called *with movement* or *with motion*. The speed of the with movement is greater for a high power minus lens than for a low power minus lens.

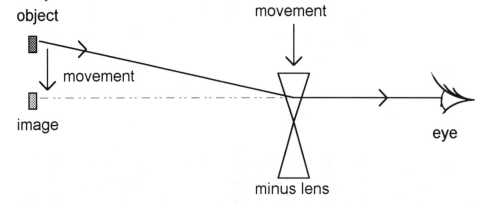

PRENTICE'S RULE

The amount of prismatic effect experienced when looking through a particular point on a lens depends on how far the point is from the optical center of the lens. This amount can be approximated using **Prentice's Rule**, one of the formulas used the most in ophthalmic optics.

$$P = \frac{d \times D}{10}$$

where P is the prism power in prism diopters,
  d is the distance from the optical center in mm,
  D is the dioptric power of the lens.

This formula may be solved for any of its variables:

$$d = \frac{P \times 10}{D}$$

or

$$D = \frac{P \times 10}{d}$$

There are a variety of forms of Prentice's rule. This book will use this form, which calls for d, the distance from the optical center, to be in mm because that is how we most commonly measure the distance in the ophthalmic lab. This formula looses accuracy for low power lenses.

EXAMPLE 1: What is the prismatic effect at a point 2mm from the optical center of a +3.00D lens?

$$P = \frac{d \times D}{10} = \frac{2 \times 3}{10} = \frac{6}{10} = \mathbf{0.6^{\Delta}}$$

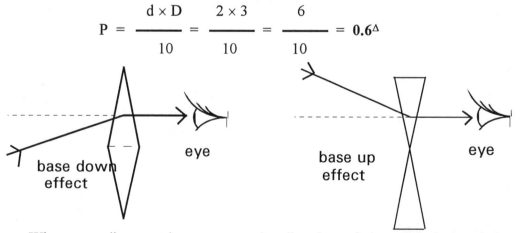

base down
effect

eye

base up
effect

eye

When recording a prism amount, the direction of the prism base relative to the wearer's eye must also be stated. A point above the optical center of a plus lens will give a base-down effect, since the base of a plus lens is at the optical center which is below the direction of gaze. A point above the optical center of a minus lens will give a base-up effect, since the base of a minus lens is away from the optical center.

EXAMPLE 2: What is the effect experienced when looking 2mm above the optical center of a +5.00D lens?

$$P = \frac{2 \times 5}{10} = \frac{10}{10} = 1.0^\Delta$$

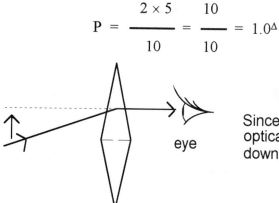

Since the person is looking above the optical center of a plus lens, the oc is down, and therefore, the prism base is down.

The answer is written **1.0$^\Delta$ BD**.

Example 3: What is the prismatic effect of looking through a point 3mm above the optical center of the Rx −3.00 −2.00 ×030?

The wearer is looking above the oc. Therefore, we need the power of the lens in the vertical or 90 degree meridian. To determine the *approximate* power on the 90th meridian we need the oblique meridian formula, pages 62-63. The axis is 30; we need 90, so we need the amount of cylinder in effect 60 degrees from the axis. Looking back at page 62, we know that 75% of the cylinder is in effect 60 degrees from the axis of the prescription. So the power on the vertical meridian is about −3.00 −1.50 = −4.50D.

Now use Prentice's rule:

$$P = \frac{d \times D}{10} = \frac{3 \times 4.50}{10} = \frac{13.50}{10} = 1.4^\Delta$$

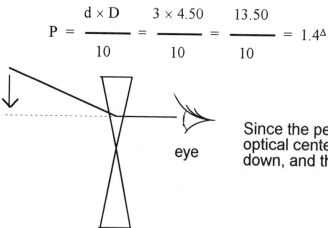

Since the person is looking above the optical center of a minus lens, the oc is down, and therefore, the prism base is up.

The answer is about **1.4$^\Delta$ BU**.

When performing calculations involving prism, always specify an amount and a base direction.

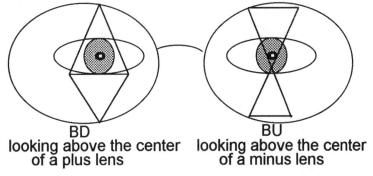

BD
looking above the center
of a plus lens

BU
looking above the center
of a minus lens

PRISMATIC EFFECT EXERCISES
(Round the answers to one-tenth prism diopter.)

1. How much prism does a wearer experience when looking 2mm below the optical center of a +4.00D lens?

2. What approximate prism would a person experience looking 4mm out on the horizontal meridian from the center of the Rx −0.50 +2.00 x030?

3. Approximately how much prism would a person experience when looking through a point 5mm toward the nasal side of a −1.00 +4.00 x075 lens?

4. What is the effect experienced when looking 5mm above the optical center of a −5.50D lens?

DETERMINING OVERALL PRISMATIC EFFECTS

When the wearer is looking through any point other than the optical centers of the lenses, there are two possible effects that the induced prism may have. One effect results from both eyes rotating the same amount and in the same direction; the other effect results from the eyes rotating different amounts or in different directions.

Causing the eyes to rotate the same amount in the same direction may cause the wearer to experience distortion. Causing the eyes to rotate different amounts or in different directions will cause, at best, discomfort. (This is sometimes diagnosed as the optical catch-all *asthenopia*, which means visual discomfort regardless of cause.) With enough difference between the eyes, *diplopia*, or *double vision*, occurs. The wearer may unconsciously suppress the vision in one eye in order to relieve the discomfort that results from diplopia. The dissociation of the eyes that causes diplopia may result in asthenopia. Sudden onset of diplopia can be caused by many things. Incorrectly made glasses is only one cause.

When there is prism induced in each of the lenses of a pair of glasses, we need to determine whether the prisms will cancel each other or compound each other.

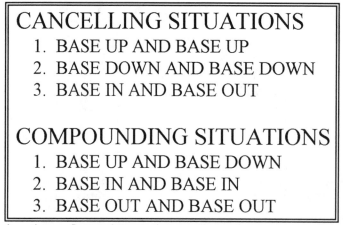

```
CANCELLING SITUATIONS
   1.  BASE UP AND BASE UP
   2.  BASE DOWN AND BASE DOWN
   3.  BASE IN AND BASE OUT

COMPOUNDING SITUATIONS
   1.  BASE UP AND BASE DOWN
   2.  BASE IN AND BASE IN
   3.  BASE OUT AND BASE OUT
```

In cancelling situations, first subtract the smaller prism amount from the larger prism amount. Then assign the prism base direction to the eye originally having the larger prism amount. In compounding situations, add the two prism amounts together to give the total effect.

EXAMPLES:

RE	LE	EFFECT	RESULTING EFFECT
2^Δ BU	3^Δ BU	cancelling	1^Δ BU LE
2^Δ BU	3^Δ BD	compounding	5^Δ BU OD or 5^Δ BD OS
2^Δ BI	2^Δ BO	cancelling	no imbalance

EXAMPLE 1: A wearer complains of headaches when using new glasses. On checking, you find that the lenses have been made with a 70mm pd, whereas the wearer's pd is 66mm. For an Rx of OU +3.00 +2.00 x060, how much prism is the wearer experiencing?

The pd is on the horizontal meridian, so we first find the approximate power on the 180 using the oblique meridian formula.

$$D_T = D_S + D_C \sin^2\alpha = +3.00 + (+2.00 \sin^2 60)$$

$$= +3.00 + (+2.00 \text{ x}0.75) = +3.00 + 1.50$$

$$D_T = +4.50D$$

The pd of the glasses is off by 4mm. We make the assumption that this error is split evenly at 2mm for each eye. (If the wearer is present or if there is a monocular pd recorded we might choose not to make that assumption.) Using Prentice's rule,

$$P = \frac{d \times D}{10} = \frac{2 \times 4.50}{10} = \frac{9.00}{10} = 0.9^\Delta$$

The lenses are plus lenses, so the base is where the optical center is. Since the glasses' pd is too big, the optical centers are out. Therefore, there is about 0.9^ΔBO for each eye, which is compounding, and the wearer is experiencing a total of about **1.8^ΔBO**.

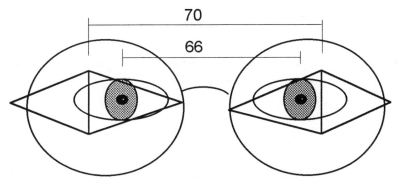

The glasses do not meet ANSI standards. The tolerance for horizontal prism is a total of 0.66^Δ, or glasses pd within 2.5mm of the wearer's pd.

EXAMPLE 2: A person has an Rx of   OD −1.00 −1.00 x045

OS −0.50 −1.00 x135

The glasses received for this person have a pd of 72mm instead of the requested 66mm. How much prism would the person experience if the glasses are dispensed, and are they within ANSI tolerance?

OD power on the horizontal meridian is about −1.50D. (Sphere + 50% cylinder.)

OS power on the horizontal meridian is about −1.00D. (Sphere + 50% cylinder.)

Each lens is off by 3mm. Using Prentice's rule,

OD

$$P = \frac{d \times D}{10} = \frac{3 \times 1.50}{10} = \frac{4.50}{10} = 0.5^\Delta \text{ BI}$$

OS

$$P = \frac{d \times D}{10} = \frac{3 \times 1.00}{10} = \frac{3.00}{10} = 0.3^\Delta \text{ BI}$$

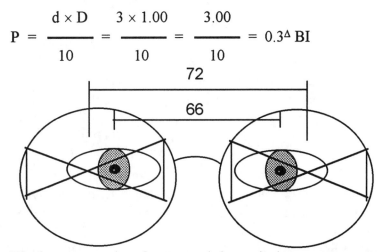

The lenses are minus lenses, and the optical centers are out. Since the base direction for minus lenses is opposite to the direction of the optical centers, the base direction is in. Total prismatic effect is about **0.8^Δ BI.**

The glasses do not meet ANSI standards.

(Round prism amount to the nearest one-tenth.)

1. About how much prism would a wearer experience if the following prescription was made to a pd of 72mm instead of 68mm as requested?

      Rx OD −0.50 −4.00 x060   OS +3.00 −4.00 x030

2. What approximate prism would a wearer experience if the following prescription was made to a pd of 70mm instead of 66mm as requested?

      Rx OD −0.50DS   OS +1.00 −4.00 x030

3. About how much prism would a wearer experience if the following prescription was made to a pd of 63mm instead of 61mm as requested?

      Rx OD −10.50 −4.00 x060   OS −13.00 −4.00 x030

4. Upon final inspection, a pair of +12.50 OU aphakic glasses show 1mm of vertical imbalance: the OD optical center is 1mm higher than the OS optical center. According to ANSI standards, these glasses are dispensable. How much vertical prism will the glasses have if the wearer's eyes are level?

5. The wearer's reading pd is 66mm, and the pre-made reading glasses pd is 60mm. If the Rx is +1.00OU, how much prism is in effect? If you dispensed them to fill an Rx of +1.00OU, would they meet ANSI standards? How much prism is in effect if the Rx and pre-made readers were +2.50OU?

ANSI STANDARDS FOR PRISM: Z80.1-1999

The position *on a single lens* where the amount of prism prescribed occurs must be no more than 1mm from where it was intended to be. If the position of the correct amount of prism is off by more than 1mm, then there must be no more than $1/3^\Delta$ error in prism at the point that should have been the prism reference point (PRP). The prism tolerance must be met whether there is prescribed prism or not. If prism is not prescribed then the prescribed prism is 0, and there must be no more than $1/3^\Delta$ of prism at the PRP.

In *a mounted pair of lenses*, the distance between the PRP's must be within 2.5mm of the requested pd, or there may be no more than $2/3^\Delta$ in total of horizontal prism error. Vertically, there must be no more than $1/3^\Delta$ of vertical imbalance, or the heights may differ by no more than 1mm. The 2.5mm rule does not apply to progressive addition lenses; they must be positioned within 1mm of the requested position, both vertically and horizontally, and each lens individually must have no more than $1/3^\Delta$ at the PRP. Prism thinning is considered prescribed prism for this tolerance test. Other styles of multifocal lenses may have the heights of the segments differ by no more than 1mm unless unequal monocular heights were specified.

The correct method of determining whether the difference between the PRP's is in tolerance is to locate and dot the position of correct prism in each lens. If the distance between these dots is within 2.5mm of the requested pd then the glasses are within ANSI tolerance. If not, dot $1/3^\Delta$ in each lens and remeasure. If the actual OC measurement was more than the pd and the new dots are less than the pd, the glasses are within ANSI tolerance. (Or, if the actual OC measurement was less than the pd and the new dots are more than the pd, the glasses are within ANSI tolerance.)

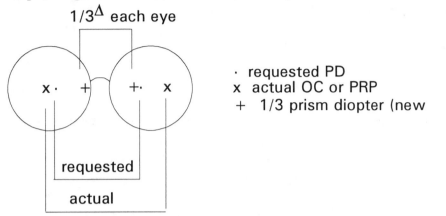

$1/3^\Delta$ each eye

· requested PD
x actual OC or PRP
+ 1/3 prism diopter (new

requested

actual

For vertical imbalance, center the *stronger* of the two lenses (on the 90th meridian) in the focimeter and dot. Move to the weaker lens without moving the stage. Read the amount of prism at this point. If the amount is less than $1/3^\Delta$, then the pair is within ANSI tolerance. If not, dot the lens, move the stage until the correct amount of prism is present, and redot. If the dots are within 1mm, the pair is within ANSI tolerance.

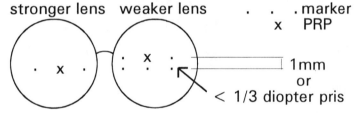

stronger lens   weaker lens   .   .   .marker
                                    x   PRP

1mm
or
< 1/3 diopter pris

SPLITTING PRISM

Occasionally, we are presented with a prescription showing prism in just one lens. In order to balance the weight of the lenses and to improve the cosmetic effect of the prism, we will **split the prism** between the two lenses. In this case, divide the amount of the prism in half. Assign one half with the base direction requested in the lens where it was prescribed. Assign the other half of the prism amount to the other eye with the base in the *compounding* direction.

EXAMPLE 1: Given the following prescription, how should the prism be split in order to even the weight of the glasses? Rx: OD pl 5^Δ BU; OS pl

Split the prisms in half, 2.5^ΔOU. Place 2.5^Δ BU in the right lens and 2.5^Δ BD in the left lens. (BU & BD compound each other.) This results in 5^Δ of vertical imbalance, with the right eye rotated down.

Order the Rx   OD pl 2.5^Δ BU
                OS pl 2.5^Δ BD

Always contact the refractionist before ordering and request permission to split the prism. There will be instances where the prescriber will not want this process to be done.

In the case where the prescriptions in the right and left eyes are very different, we may want to split the prism unequally in the effort to equalize weight and thickness. This will require determining the edge thicknesses for the lens and the prism. These thickness formulas are in Section V of this book.

EXAMPLE 2: Given the prescription OD pl 5$^\Delta$BU
OS pl 3$^\Delta$BI
how could the prism be split to even the weight and thickness of the glasses?

The vertical prism would be split 2.5D BU in the right lens and 2.5D BD in the left lens. The horizontal prism would be split 1.5$^\Delta$BI OU. The result would be:

OD pl 2.5$^\Delta$ BU & 1.5$^\Delta$ BI
OS pl 2.5$^\Delta$ BD & 1.5$^\Delta$ BI

On pages 98-103 is a discussion of how to fabricate this prism.

SPLITTING THE PRISM EXERCISES
If the prescription form indicates that splitting the prism is acceptable, what prism would you order for the following Rx's?

1. OD +2.50DS 3$^\Delta$BU
   OS +2.50DS

2. OD −5.00
   OS −5.00 4$^\Delta$BI

3. OD −1.00 −1.00 x180 3$^\Delta$BO
   OS −1.00 −1.00 x180

4. OD +1.50 −0.50 x090
   OS +1.00   5$^\Delta$BD

EXCESSIVE OR UNWANTED PRISM
It is possible for the pd of the completed glasses to be correct, and the wearer to still indicate that something "seems" or "feels" wrong. This could be the result of the optical centers being offset equal amounts, resulting in equal amounts of prism in each eye that cancel each other. For example, if the optical centers are 5mm below the wearer's pupils with a prescription of −4.00DS OU, both lenses would have 2$^\Delta$ of BU prism. Another example might be if the wearer's monocular pd's were 28/32 for a +6.00DS OU prescription, but the optical centers were inset equal amounts, the right lens would have 1.2$^\Delta$ BO and the left lens would have 1.2$^\Delta$ BI. (We will discuss correcting the first situation using pantoscopic tilt in Section VI.)

EXCESSIVE OR UNWANTED BASE DOWN PRISM

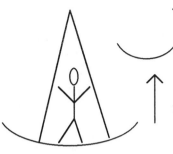

1. Causes the floor or other horizontal expanse to seem concave. The wearer feels like the floor is the bottom of a bowl.

2. Makes people and vertical objects seem taller.

3. Makes the floor seem to slant uphill.

EXCESSIVE OR UNWANTED BASE UP PRISM

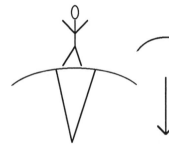

1. Causes the floor or other horizontal expanse to seem convex. The wearer feels like the floor is a pitcher's mound.

2. Makes people and vertical objects seem shorter.

3. Makes the floor seem to slant downhill.

EXCESSIVE BASE OUT OR BASE IN PRISM

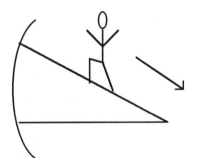

Causes the wearer to see horizontal objects, such as a table or floor, to be sloped. The side with the base appears higher than the side with the apex.

IMAGE JUMP

New bifocal wearers sometimes complain that the object they look down at moves, or jumps, as the eye rotates down into the bifocal segment. Experienced bifocal wearers who change bifocal style may also have this complaint. This is called *image jump* and is a function of the position of the segment optical center and the add power of the segment

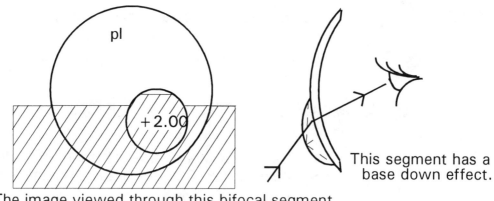

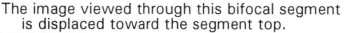

This segment has a base down effect.

The image viewed through this bifocal segment is displaced toward the segment top.

When the wearer looks through the top of a 22mm round bifocal segment, the person is looking through a point that is 11mm from the OC of the segment. For an add of +2.00D, the approximate prismatic effect can be found using Prentice's rule.

$$ P = \frac{d \times D}{10} = \frac{11 \times 2.00}{10} = 2.2^\Delta \, BD $$

There is a 2.2^Δ image jump resulting from the direction of gaze traveling into the top of the bifocal segment. Note that this is independent of the power of the distance prescription. The amount of prism experienced through the distance portion does not undergo a noticeable sudden increase or decrease over the short distance from just above the segment top to just inside the segment.

As a general rule of thumb, the OC of a segment is about

> 11 mm from the top of a round 22
>
> 4-6 mm from the top of most FT or ST (assume 5 mm if not told otherwise)
>
> 19 mm from the top of an Ultex A and AX
>
> 0 mm from the top of an executive (or SL) and a progressive

IMAGE JUMP EXERCISES
(Round to one-tenth prism diopter.)

1. What image jump is present for the Rx

      OD   −1.00DS add +2.50 OU

      OS   −1.50DS   made with FT28s?

2. What image jump is present for the Rx

      OD   −1.00DS add +2.50 OU

      OS   −1.50DS   made with executives?

3. What image jump is present on the Rx

      OD   −1.00DS add +2.25

      OS   −1.50DS add +3.00 made with round 22?

ANISOMETROPIA

Anisometropia is defined as the condition where the eyes have different refractive errors. Anisometropia requires only that there be a difference in amount, not necessarily in type. The *a-* or *an-* suffix on a word generally means "not"; so *isometropia* is a condition where the eyes have the same refractive error or no error at all. *Antimetropia* is a special case of anisometropia: it is the condition where the prescriptions have different signs.

EXAMPLES

	1.	2.	3.	4.
OD	−3.00D	−1.00D	+1.00D	+2.25D
OS	−5.00D	+1.00D	+5.00D	+2.25D
	anisometropia	anisometropia	anisometropia	isometropia
		antimetropia		

Textbooks generally do not specify how much difference is needed in order to say that the person is anisometropic. If the person is experiencing a problem that is the result of a difference in magnification or prismatic effect, then the person is anisometropic, or has anisometropia.

Differences in magnification result in a lack of fusion. Lenses designed to minimize this problem are called iseikonic lenses. We will discuss these lenses in Spectacle Magnification in Section VI.

Differences in prismatic effect, like differences in magnification, will result in a lack of fusion.

VERTICAL IMBALANCE

Whenever we look through a point other than the optical center of our lenses, we experience a prismatic effect. This is particularly true when the wearer is forced to look through the bifocal segment of the lens in order to read. The amount of prismatic effect will depend on the prescription and how far away from the optical center the wearer is looking. If each eye has a different prescription, vertical imbalance will be present. If there is enough imbalance, the person may have *diplopia* (double vision), or may suppress one eye.

The wearer can avoid the vertical imbalance when wearing single vision lenses by adjusting the position of the head to always look through the optical center. A person wearing bifocals cannot avoid the imbalance, as this person must look through the bifocal in order to read. We have several ways to offset this imbalance. We can dispense *two pair of single vision glasses*, one for distance and one for reading. We can use **different segment styles**, giving different amounts of segment-induced prism at the reading level. We can use special *prism-controlled segments*, which are discussed in dispensing texts such as Brooks & Borish *Systems for Ophthalmic Dispensing*. Or we can use **bicentric grinding**, or **slab-off**. The name bicentric grinding comes from the fact that we are literally creating two distance optical centers on the same lens without changing the distance prescription.

CALCULATING VERTICAL IMBALANCE

When bifocals are made with identical style, shape, size, and power segments, any vertical imbalance will be due to the distance prescription only. To determine how much imbalance is present, it is necessary to know what the approximate power on the 90th meridian is and how far from the distance optical center the wearer will be looking.

EXAMPLE: Calculate the vertical imbalance present at a reading position 10mm below the distance optical center for the following Rx:

OD −1.00D   OS −4.00D   ADD +2.00D OU

RIGHT EYE   LEFT EYE
d = 10mm   d = 10mm
D = −1.00D   D = −4.00D

$$P = \frac{d \times D}{10}$$ $$P = \frac{d \times D}{10}$$

$$P = \frac{10 \times 1.00}{10}$$ $$P = \frac{10 \times 4.00}{10}$$

P = 1$^\triangle$ BD   **P = 4$^\triangle$ BD**

The vertical imbalance is the combination of the prism in the two lenses. In this case, the prisms are cancelling, and the vertical imbalance is **3$^\triangle$ BD** in the left eye.

USING TWO DIFFERENT SEGMENT STYLES

Sometimes we can use unlike segments to cancel the imbalance at the reading level. Look back at the drawing on page 88 showing the image jump for a 22mm round bifocal. The upper half of the round segment contains base down prism. An executive or progressive addition lens (PAL) style bifocal has the OC of the segment at the top of the segment, so the prism induced by the executive or PAL segment is BU. Since a flat top 22, 28 or 35 usually has the segment OC about 5mm below the top of the segment, the wearer may be looking through either BU or BD induced by the segment, depending on the reading level.

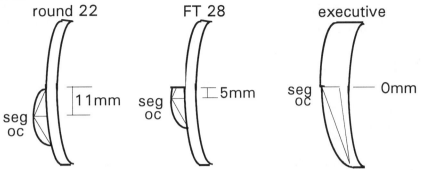

round 22   FT 28   executive

seg
oc |11mm   seg   I5mm   seg   ─── 0mm
              oc   oc

Suppose the wearer has a +2.50 add and 1.5△ of imbalance at the reading level, which is 4mm below the top of the segment. 4mm below the top of the segment is 7mm above the OC of the round 22, 1mm above the OC of the FT28, and 4mm below the OC of the executive. Using Prentice's rule and +2.50 adds, to determine the induced prism in the segment, we have:

	round 22	FT28	executive/PAL
add (D)	+2.50	+2.50	+2.50
d	7mm	1mm	4mm
P△	1.8△ BD	0.3△ BD	1.0△ BU

We can make use of these differing amounts of prism induced by different segment styles to minimize the vertical imbalance induced by the distance prescription. Placing a round segment over the eye with the most BU or the least BD in the distance portion and placing a FT28 over the eye with the least BU or the most BD in the distance portion would induce a 1.5△ imbalance that is opposite to the imbalance induced by the distance prescription.

We can use Prentice's rule to determine how much difference there should be between the segment OC's to neutralize the distance induced imbalance. This technique assumes that the segments will have the same add power.

$$ d = \frac{P \times 10}{D} $$

where P is the imbalance from the distance Rx at the reading level,
D is the add power of the Rx,
d is the difference between the segment OC placements.

Lost?

EXAMPLE 1: The prescription is   −3.00DS   add +1.50 OU
                                    −1.50DS

The reading level is 8mm below OC, and the segments are to be set 5mm below OC. What segments should we use to eliminate most of the imbalance at the reading level?

Step 1. First determine the imbalance at the reading level due to the distance prescription.

OD −3.00D   OS −1.50D   ADD +1.50D OU

RIGHT EYE   LEFT EYE

d = 8mm   d = 8mm

D = −3.00D   D = −1.50D

$$P = \frac{d \times D}{10}$$ $$P = \frac{d \times D}{10}$$

$$P = \frac{8 \times 3.00}{10}$$ $$P = \frac{8 \times 1.25}{10}$$

$$P = 2.4^\Delta \text{ BD}$$ $$P = 1.2^\Delta \text{ BD}$$

The vertical imbalance at the reading level is the difference between the prism amounts for the two lenses, or **1.2^Δ BD OD**.

Step 2. Determine the difference needed between the OC's of the segments to compensate for the distance imbalance.

Using 1.2^Δ for P and +1.50D (the add power) for D in Prentice's rule, we get

$$d = \frac{P \times 10}{D} = \frac{1.2 \times 10}{1.50} = 8 \text{ mm, the needed difference between seg OC's.}$$

Step 3. Decide what segments will give the needed compensating imbalance.

The difference between FT28 OC (5mm) and round 22 OC (11mm) is close to the difference computed. The round 22 will induce more BD that the FT28 will. We want to either increase the BD effect of the left eye distance prescription or decrease the BD effect of the right eye distance prescription. Placing the FT28 in the right lens and the round 22 in the left lens will help eliminate the imbalance at the reading level. The remaining imbalance should be small enough to cause little problem.

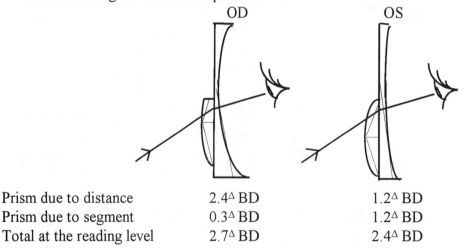

OD   OS

	OD	OS
Prism due to distance	2.4^Δ BD	1.2^Δ BD
Prism due to segment	0.3^Δ BD	1.2^Δ BD
Total at the reading level	2.7^Δ BD	2.4^Δ BD

The table below gives the number of mm difference between the segments. In example 1, we determined that we needed about 8mm difference between the segments. The table below tells us that we can have a 6mm difference by using FT28 and a round 22 in the OS, or we can use an executive and a round 22. The lens with the least minus power is the OS. In the pair FT28 and round 22, the lowest OC is the round 22, so it goes on the OS. In the pair executive and round 22, the round 22 is also the one with the lowest OC, so it goes on the OS. A FT25 in the right lens and a round 22 in the left lens will probably look best.

SEGMENT DIFFERENCES in mm				
OD Segment	OS Segment			
	round 22	FT	executive/PAL	ultex
round 22	0	6	11	8
FT 25/28/35	6	0	5	14
executive/PAL	11	5	0	19
ultex	8	14	19	0

Rule for where to put the segments:

> **Place the segment with the lowest OC placement on the lens with the most plus power or the lens with the least minus power in the vertical meridian.**

EXAMPLE 2: The prescription reads OD +1.25DS, OS pl, add +2.50 OU. The glasses have FT28's with segment drop of 5mm, and the reading level is 9mm. If the wearer is experiencing problems fusing when reading, what segment change might you make?

OD +1.25D   OS pl   ADD +2.00D OU
RIGHT EYE   LEFT EYE
d = 9mm   d = 9mm
D = +1.25D   D = 0D

$$P = \frac{d \times D}{10}$$ $$P = \frac{d \times D}{10}$$

$$P = \frac{9 \times 1.25}{10}$$ $$P = \frac{9 \times 0}{10}$$

$$P = 1.1^\Delta \, BU$$ $$P = 0^\Delta$$

The imbalance at the reading level is 1.1^ΔBU in the right eye. Using Prentice's rule,

$$d = \frac{P \times 10}{D} = \frac{1.1 \times 10}{2.5} = 4mm, \text{ the needed difference between seg OC's.}$$

We need BD in the right eye, or BU in the left eye. The table tells us that we can get 5mm difference by replacing one of the FT28's with an executive or PAL. The FT28 has the lower OC placement, and the lens with the most plus/least minus is the OD. So the left lens could be changed to an executive or PAL.

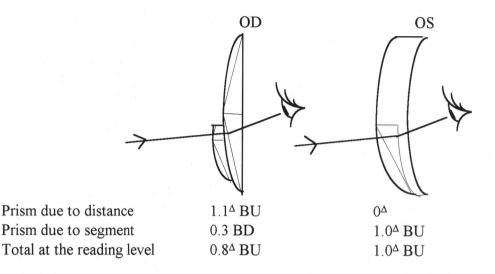

	OD	OS
Prism due to distance	1.1$^\Delta$ BU	0$^\Delta$
Prism due to segment	0.3 BD	1.0$^\Delta$ BU
Total at the reading level	0.8$^\Delta$ BU	1.0$^\Delta$ BU

TWO DIFFERENT SEGMENT STYLE EXERCISE

1. The prescription reads OD −0.50DS OS +0.75DS, add +2.00OU. The reading level is 10mm below OC, and the segments are 7mm below OC. What segments could you use to reduce the imbalance at the reading level?

BICENTRIC GRINDING OR SLAB-OFF

Bicentric grinding or *slab-off* is the process used to change the amount of prism in the reading portion of the lens, while not affecting the prism in the distance portion of the lens. Slab-off results in base up prism in the reading area. It is ground on the lens that has the weakest plus or strongest minus power on the 90th meridian.

Reverse slab-off is molded on the convex side of plastic lenses and is the exact opposite of regular slab-off. Reverse slab-off results in base down prism in the reading area and it is molded on the lens with the strongest plus or weakest minus power on the 90th meridian.

	SLAB-OFF	REVERSE SLAB-OFF
two minus lenses	highest minus	lowest minus
two plus lenses	lowest plus	highest plus
one plus, one minus	the minus lens	the plus lens

Usually, slab-off is only ordered if the imbalance results in 1.5$^\Delta$ or more. The lens reference book published by FRAMES currently lists two companies who can supply a reverse slab-off of 1.0$^\Delta$. When calculating the amount of prism, remember that the result is an approximation. The direction of gaze is actually in as well as down, and the oblique meridian formula results in an approximation of the power. The technique shown below results in a reasonable estimate of the vertical imbalance that needs to be corrected in order for the wearer to read comfortably.

EXAMPLE: What is the approximate vertical imbalance at a reading level of 10mm, and what slab-off could be ordered for the following prescription?

OD −1.00 −2.00 x090   ADD +2.50D OU

OS +1.00 −1.00 x060

Step 1. Find the distance power on the vertical meridian for each lens.

The right eye power on the 90th meridian is −1.00D. The left eye power in the 90th meridian is about +0.75D. (This is found using the oblique meridian formula, pages 62-63.)

Step 2. Find the prismatic effect at the reading level for each lens.

PRISMATIC EFFECT when looking 10mm below the optical center:

RIGHT EYE   LEFT EYE

$$P = \frac{10 \times 1.00}{10} \qquad\qquad P = \frac{10 \times 0.75}{10}$$

$P = 1^\Delta$ BD $P = 0.8^\Delta$ BU

Step 3. Determine the total imbalance between the two prescriptions.

The prism amounts are compounding, so the vertical imbalance in this pair is about **OD 1.8$^\Delta$ BD** or **OS 1.8$^\Delta$ BU**. Use a 1.75$^\Delta$ slab-off on the right lens or a 1.75$^\Delta$ reverse slab-off on the left lens.

SLAB-OFF EXERCISES

(Round the prism amounts to one-tenth diopter.)

1. What is the approximate vertical imbalance at a reading level of 8mm for the following prescription? What slab-off could be ordered, and in which lens?

OD −2.00 −4.00 x030   ADD +3.00D

OS −1.00 −1.00 x030

2. Compute the approximate vertical imbalance at a reading level of 7mm for the following prescription. What slab-off could be ordered, and in which lens?

OD +7.50 −1.50 x015   Add +2.50D

OS +3.50 −2.00 x165

3. What is the approximate vertical imbalance at a reading level of 10mm for the following prescription? What slab-off could be ordered, and in which lens?

OD +1.00 −4.00 x060   ADD +2.00D

OS −2.00 −1.00 x030

VERTICAL IMBALANCE FOR UNLIKE ADD POWERS

The situation becomes a little more complex when the bifocals adds are of different powers, or the segments are in different positions, are different sizes, or are different styles. In this case, we cannot stop with just the imbalance generated by the different distance powers. Now, we can determine how far below the top of the segment the reading level is and how far the segment optical center is from that reading level, and add the reading imbalance to the distance imbalance. The steps are:

1. Determine the imbalance from the distance portion of the lenses.
2. Determine the distance that the reading level is with respect to the OC's of the segments.
3. Determine the imbalance from the segments.
4. Combine the imbalances from distance and segment to give the total imbalance present at the reading level.

EXAMPLE 1: Given the prescription:

OD pl   ADD +2.50
OS +2.00   ADD +1.50

The reading level is 9mm below OC, and the round 22 bifocal segments are set at 5mm below OC. What bicentric grind should be ordered?

1. The vertical imbalance for the distance Rx is OS 1.8$^\Delta$BU.
2. Refer back to the discussion of image jump, pages 88-89, for the approximate position of the segment optical center in the common bifocal styles. For this example the drop is 5mm and the reading level is 9mm, so the reading level is 4mm below the top of the segment, and is therefore 7mm from the OC of the segment.

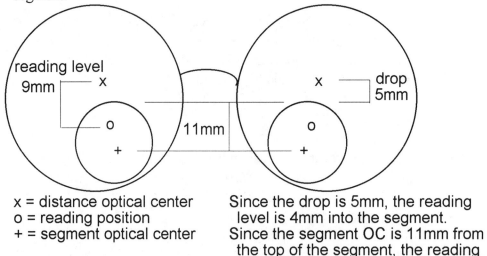

x = distance optical center
o = reading position
+ = segment optical center

Since the drop is 5mm, the reading level is 4mm into the segment. Since the segment OC is 11mm from the top of the segment, the reading level is 7mm above the segment OC.

3. Since the wearer is looking 7mm above the optical centers in these glasses, the prism resulting from the segment for the right eye is (7)(2.50)/10 = 1.75$^\Delta$ BD, and for the left eye is (7)(1.50)/10 = 1.05$^\Delta$BD, for a total imbalance from the segments of 0.7BD OD.
4. The vertical imbalance for the distance is OS 1.8$^\Delta$BU, and for the segments is OD 0.7$^\Delta$BD. **The prisms are compounding, and result in about 2.5$^\Delta$BU OS or 2.5$^\Delta$BD OD.** Since the left eye is the highest plus for the distance Rx, we could do either reverse slab-off of 2.5$^\Delta$ in the left lens or regular slab-off of 2.5$^\Delta$ in the right lens.

EXAMPLE 2: Rx   OD −1.50 −2.00 x090   ADD +2.50
                        OS −4.00 − 1.00 x045   ADD +2.00

The wearer has ST28's. Reading level is 8mm below OC, seg drop is 5mm. What bicentric grind should be ordered?

1. Determine the lens distance power on the 90th meridian, the prism amount for the distance Rx at the reading level, and the total imbalance.

   OD power on the 90th is −1.50; prism amount is 1.2△ BD.
   OS power on the 90th is about −4.50; prism amount is 3.6△ BD.
   Total imbalance for the distance Rx is about 2.4△ BD OS.

2. Determine how far the reading level is from the segment optical center.

   The reading level is 3mm below the top of the segment. The segment OC is 5mm below the top of the segment. Therefore, the reading level is 2mm from the optical center of the segment.

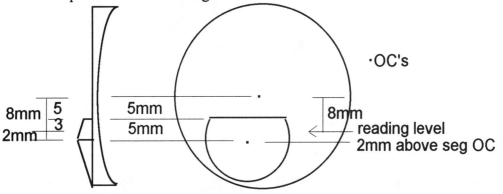

3. Determine the imbalance induced by the segments.

   OD power in the segment is +2.50; prism amount is (2)(2.50)/10 = 0.5△ BD.
   OS power in the segment is +2.00; prism amount is (2)(2.00)/10 = 0.4△ BD.
   Total imbalance for the segment is 0.1△ BD OD.

4. Combine the two total imbalances.

   Combining 2.4△ BD OS with 0.1△ BD OD results in about 2.3△ BD OS. (They are cancelling.)

Use the combined imbalance for the amount of slab-off, and assign it to the high minus/low plus for regular slab-off or high plus/low minus for reverse slab-off.

Request about 2.3△ slab-off in the OS or 2.3△ reverse slab-off in the OD.

Note: The reading position is not actually on the 90th meridian. The eyes converge as they are lowered to read, so we should be computing the prism amount about 2mm in from the OC and 8mm below it. Using the resultant prism calculations that we will cover next we could find this exact answer. However, the answer that we get with the method above is adequate for determining bicentric grind.

Note: Slab-off can be ground in any prism amount, but reverse slab-off is molded on to the front surface of the lens, so the choices are limited. This is not a problem, as the wearer will unconsciously adjust the reading level to where vision is comfortable.

RESULTANT PRISM

Prescribed prism is rarely just up, down, in, or out. Instead, the Rx may look like this:

    OD   pl   3$^\Delta$BU & 5$^\Delta$ BI

    OS   pl   3$^\Delta$BD & 5$^\Delta$BI

What should you look for in the focimeter (or lensometer) when marking up the glasses? We call what will be seen in the focimeter the ***resultant prism***. Or you may be neutralizing a pair of glasses and see the following in the focimeter. How would you write this in horizontal and vertical components? We call this ***resolving the prism.***

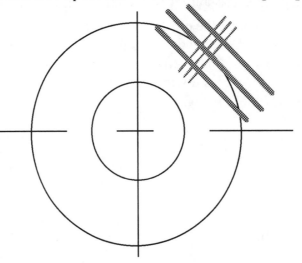

BASE DIRECTION AND PRISM AXIS

When looking at a pair of glasses from the convex side, we might imagine the lenses split into four quadrants.

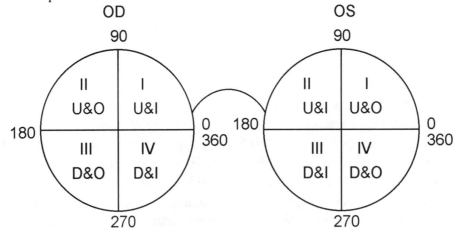

Quadrants I and II are always "UP", and quadrants III and IV are always "DOWN". II and III are on the left, and I and IV are on the right. Which two are "IN" or "OUT" depends on which eye the lens is for. (IN is toward the nose. OUT is toward the temple.)

    Quadrant I has base direction UP and IN for the right eye, or UP and OUT for the left eye. The direction of the prism base is between 0 and 90 degrees.

Quadrant II has base direction UP and OUT for the right eye, or UP and IN for the left eye. The direction of the prism base is between 90 and 180 degrees.

Quadrant III has base direction DOWN and OUT for the right eye, or DOWN and IN for the left eye. The direction of the prism base is between 180 and 270 degrees.

Quadrant IV has base direction DOWN and IN for the right eye, or DOWN and OUT for the left eye. The direction of the prism base is between 270 and 360 degrees.

Prism base down and out is very different from prism base up and in, so we use 180-360 degrees for down. When discussing cylinder axis, no distinction is made between up and down because it is not necessary.

EXAMPLE:

    OD pl 3ᐃBU & 5ᐃ BI

    OS pl 3ᐃBD & 5ᐃBI

From the second diagram on page 98, we see that the OD prism is in quadrant I, and the OS prism is in quadrant III. Therefore, we can expect the direction of the prism base to be between 0 and 90 degrees for the right eye, and between 180 and 270 degrees for the left eye. Look first at the right eye.

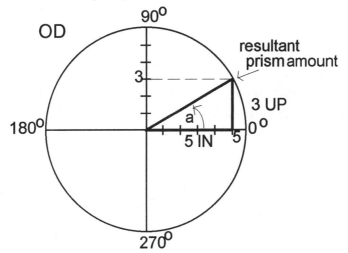

Do you see the right triangle made by the horizontal and vertical sides of the prescribed prism? The angle a in the diagram tells us where the prism is located within quadrant I and is the angle that the longest side of the triangle makes with the horizontal axis of the lens. The resultant amount of the prism is the length of the longest side of the triangle. (A right triangle is a triangle with one 90 degree angle. The longest side is called the hypotenuse and is opposite the right angle in the triangle.)

If we use P for the amount of the resultant prism, H for the amount of the horizontal prism, and V for the amount of the vertical prism, then (using Pythagoras' theorem)

$$P^2 = H^2 + V^2$$

and the angle a shown in the diagram has

$$\tan a = V / H$$

In this example, H = 5, V = 3, $P^2 = 5^2 + 3^2 = 34$, and $P = \sqrt{34} = 5.8^\Delta$,

      tan a = 3/5 = 0.6, and a = 31°

31° is between 0 and 90, which is what we wanted, so the resultant prism is **5.8$^\Delta$@ 031**, or **5.8$^\Delta$ BU&I @ 031°**. In the focimeter, the target will look like:

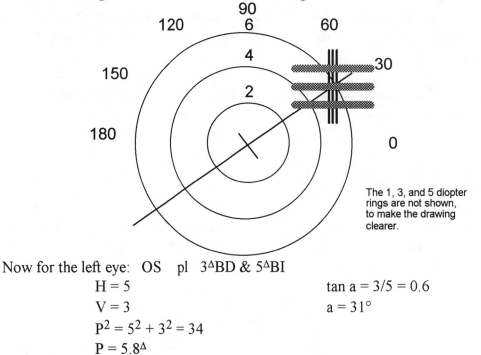

The 1, 3, and 5 diopter rings are not shown, to make the drawing clearer.

Now for the left eye: OS pl 3$^\Delta$BD & 5$^\Delta$BI

    H = 5   tan a = 3/5 = 0.6

    V = 3   a = 31°

    $P^2 = 5^2 + 3^2 = 34$

    $P = 5.8^\Delta$

But this time, we needed the axis to be between 180 and 270 since the prism is in quadrant III. Here is what the prism looks like:

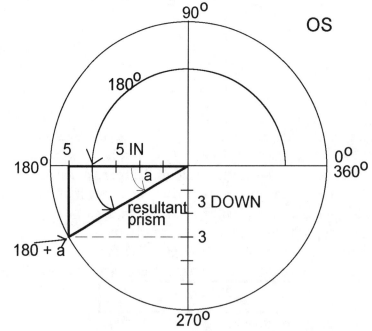

To find the correct angle, we add 180 degrees to the 31 from the formula. So the resultant prism is **5.8$^\Delta$@ 211**.

Most focimeters only show the axis notation between 0 and 180, so we cannot read the axis directly at 211 degrees. Therefore, sometimes we show prism axis that should have been between 180 and 360 as the equivalent amount between 0 and 180 degrees. When the base direction is DOWN subtract 180 degrees from the axis for the prism. In the example above, the answer may be written **5.8$^\Delta$ BD&I @ 031°**. Notice that we have included the directions BD&I this time. When the prism was written 5.8$^\Delta$ @ 211°, there was no doubt where the base was: it was in the third quadrant. In the notation 5.8$^\Delta$ BD&I @ 031°, if we omit the BD&I, the base would be in the first quadrant instead of the third quadrant, and the wearer would have the prism in the worst possible wrong direction!

When we leave the base direction (BD&I or BU&O, etc.) off, we force the person reading the prescription to assume that we are giving the actual direction with the axis. In other words, if the base were in the third or fourth quadrant, the axis would be between 180 and 360 degrees. We call this the *360 degree notation*. The prism amount 1$^\Delta$ @ 028 means the prism is in the first quadrant. It cannot be in the third quadrant. The prism amount 1$^\Delta$ @ 135 is in the second quadrant; it cannot be in the fourth quadrant. Likewise, the prism amount 1$^\Delta$ @ 240 is in the third quadrant, and the prism amount 1$^\Delta$ @ 328 is in the fourth quadrant. This is 360 degree notation because we are using all of the 360 degrees in the circle.

On the other hand, if we state the base direction using BU, BD, BI and BO, we can use the more familiar *180 degree notation*, where we do not use any degrees above 180. For the right lens the prism 1$^\Delta$ @ 028 becomes 1$^\Delta$ BU&I @ 028; 1$^\Delta$ @ 135 becomes 1$^\Delta$ BU&O @ 135; 1$^\Delta$ @ 240 becomes 1$^\Delta$ BD&O @ 060 (because 240 − 180 = 060); 1$^\Delta$ @ 328 becomes 1$^\Delta$ BD&I @ 148 (because 328 − 180 = 148). Notice that because the upper half of the lens is always between 0 and 180 degrees, the two notations have the same axis in quadrant I and II. In the lower half of the lens, the axis for the two notations differ by exactly 180 degrees.

Remember: the base direction for prism is not like the cylinder notation, where what happens in the top of the lens also happens in the bottom of the lens. We are talking about prism base direction, where a base at 90 degrees is very different from a base at 270 degrees.

EXAMPLES:
   a. 1$^\Delta$ BD&O @ 045 = 1$^\Delta$ @ 225 (Note: This is OD. WHY?)
   b. 3.5$^\Delta$ BD&I @ 120 = 3.5$^\Delta$ @ 300 (Note: Which eye?)
   c. OD 4.25$^\Delta$ @ 275 = 4.25$^\Delta$ BD&I @ 095
   d. OS 2$^\Delta$ @ 193 = 2$^\Delta$ BD&I @ 013
   e. 1.5$^\Delta$ BU&O @040 = 1.5$^\Delta$ @ 040 (Why are the angles the same? Which eye is this?)

RULES FOR THE ANGLE, after using the formula:

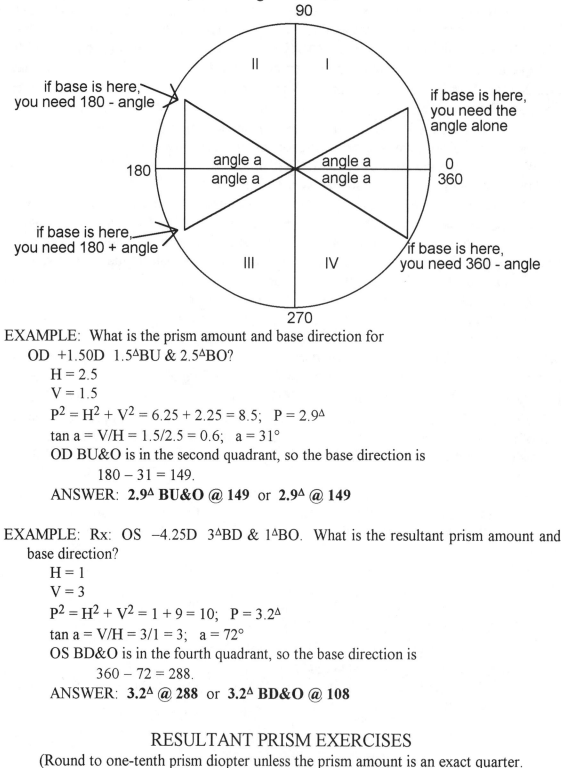

EXAMPLE: What is the prism amount and base direction for

OD +1.50D 1.5^ΔBU & 2.5^ΔBO?

     H = 2.5

     V = 1.5

     $P^2 = H^2 + V^2 = 6.25 + 2.25 = 8.5$; $P = 2.9^\Delta$

     tan a = V/H = 1.5/2.5 = 0.6; a = 31°

     OD BU&O is in the second quadrant, so the base direction is

          180 − 31 = 149.

     ANSWER: **2.9^Δ BU&O @ 149** or **2.9^Δ @ 149**

EXAMPLE: Rx: OS −4.25D 3^ΔBD & 1^ΔBO. What is the resultant prism amount and base direction?

     H = 1

     V = 3

     $P^2 = H^2 + V^2 = 1 + 9 = 10$; $P = 3.2^\Delta$

     tan a = V/H = 3/1 = 3; a = 72°

     OS BD&O is in the fourth quadrant, so the base direction is

          360 − 72 = 288.

     ANSWER: **3.2^Δ @ 288** or **3.2^Δ BD&O @ 108**

RESULTANT PRISM EXERCISES

(Round to one-tenth prism diopter unless the prism amount is an exact quarter.
Round base direction to whole angles.)

1. What are the prism amount and base direction for:

     OD +1.00D 2.25^ΔBU & 2.25^ΔBI?

2. OS −0.50 −0.50 x090 1.0ᐃBI & 2.0ᐃBU.   What is the amount and base direction of the resultant prism?

3. If the prism prescribed is 4ᐃBD & 3ᐃBI for the right eye, where would the resultant prism be located in the focimeter target?

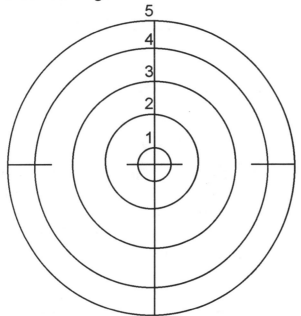

4.   If the prism prescribed is 2ᐃBU & 3ᐃBO for the left eye, where would the resultant prism be located in the focimeter target above?

RESOLVING PRISM

The formulas for resolving a prism into vertical and horizontal parts are

$$V = (P)(\sin a)$$
$$H = (P)(\cos a)$$

where P = the amount of the resultant prism,
          V = the vertical component,
          H = the horizontal component.

EXAMPLE 1: The prism found in the focimeter for a pair of glasses is 2.0ᐃ @ 045, and the lens is a right lens. Resolve this prism into its component parts.

On the diagram on the next page, the long side P of the triangle is 2.0, and the angle a that the prism makes with the axis is 45 degrees. 45° is quadrant I, which is U and I for the right lens.

   V = (P)(sin a) = (2.0)(sin 45) = (2)(0.707) = 1.4ᐃ BU, since V is vertical.

   H = (P)(cos a) = (2.0)(cos 45) = (2)(0.707) = 1.4ᐃ BI since H is horizontal.

The prism resolves to 1.4ᐃ BI & 1.4ᐃ BU.

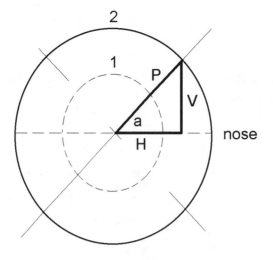

EXAMPLE 2: Resolve 4$^\Delta$ BU&I @ 105° into its component parts. Which eye is it for?
  P = 4. (In these formulas, ignore the sign of the sine and cosine functions.)
  V = (P)(sin a) = (4)(sin 105) = (4)(0.966) = 3.9$^\Delta$ BU.
  H = (P)(cos a) = (4)(cos 105) = (4)(0.259) = 1.0$^\Delta$ BI.
  The answer is 3.9$^\Delta$ BU & 1.0$^\Delta$ BI.   105 degrees is in quadrant II;   BU&I is in
  quadrant II only for the left lens.

EXAMPLE 3:   Resolve OD 3.5$^\Delta$ @ 300° into its component parts. (In these formulas,
  ignore the sign of the sine and cosine functions.)
  P = 3.5
  300° is in quadrant IV, which is BD&I for the right lens.
  V = (P)(sin a) = (3.5)(sin 300) = (3.5)(0.866) = 3.0$^\Delta$ BD.
  H = (P)(cos a) = (3.5)(cos 300) = (3.5)(0.5) = 1.8$^\Delta$ BI.
    The answer is 3.0$^\Delta$ BD & 1.8$^\Delta$ BI.

RESOLVING PRISM EXERCISES
(Round to one-tenth prism diopter unless the prism amount is an exact quarter.
Round base direction to whole angles.)

1. Resolve OD 2.25$^\Delta$ @ 255° into its component parts.

2. Resolve OS 4.25$^\Delta$ BD&I @ 45° into its component parts.

3.   What are the component parts of the prism shown on the next page? This is a left
lens. (The target is 1/3 of the way between the two circles.)

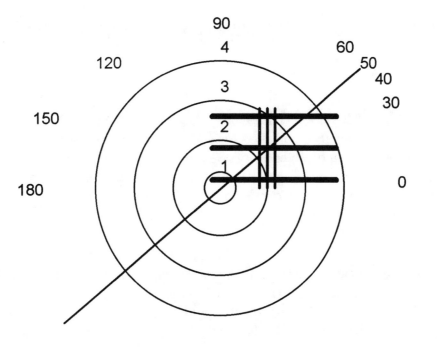

SECTION V: SURFACING AND FINISHING

LENS AND FRAME MEASUREMENTS

When marking a lens to be blocked for surfacing, non-computerized systems require determining where the optical center of the lens will be. We may need to know the amount of *decentration per lens* and the *minimum blank size*. In order to compute either of these values, we first need a consistent way of measuring the lens. There are two measurement systems currently in use.

BOXING SYSTEM

In the boxing system, a rectangle is drawn around each lens, allowing us to find the **geometrical center** of the lens. The geometrical center is half-way from the top to the bottom of the lens, and half-way from the right side to the left side of the lens. The horizontal length of the rectangle is called the *eyesize*, or *A measurement*, and the vertical length of the rectangle is called the *depth*, or *B measurement.*

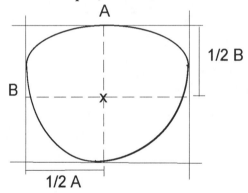

x is the geometric center of the lens

After a pair of lenses have been mounted in a frame, there is also a **distance between lenses**, or **DBL.**

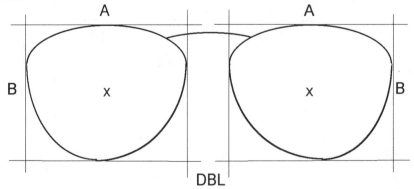

Note that the DBL is the measurement between the lenses, not necessarily the length of the bridge of the frame.

On a rimless frame or a frame with thin metal wires, the DBL can be measured directly from the lenses or from the frame. It is the smallest distance between lenses. On the thick frame below, the edge of the lens is (or eventually will be) inside the thickness of the frame. In this case, we make the assumption that the lens bevel will be 1/2mm inside the frame. Therefore, the DBL is measured from the inside of one eyewire to the inside of the other eyewire, and then 1 mm is subtracted from the measurement. Likewise, the desired A and B measurements are taken from the inside of the eyewire, and 1mm is *added* to them.

This distance plus 1/2mm on each side is the A measurement. So we add 1mm to the measurement.

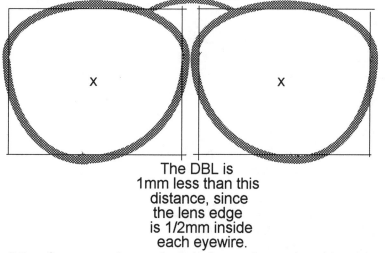

This distance plus 1/2mm inside the top eyewire and 1/2mm inside the bottom eyewire is the B measurement. Add 1mm to the measurement.

The DBL is 1mm less than this distance, since the lens edge is 1/2mm inside each eyewire.

Manufacturers who mark their frame sizes using this system use a small box between the A and DBL: "52 ☐ 18" means a frame with an A measurement of 52 and a DBL of 18, using the boxing system.

DATUM SYSTEM

Many manufacturers use the Datum system instead of the boxing system to show the measurements of the frame. In the Datum system, we draw a horizontal line half-way between the top and bottom of the lens. The width of the lens at this point is the *datum* or *D measurement*. The distance between the lenses at this point is the DBL. The datum system frequently gives a smaller eyesize and a larger DBL than the boxing system does.

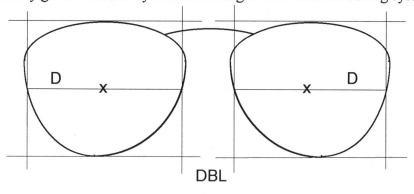

DBL

FRAME PD

If no prism was prescribed, then the completed glasses should have the optical centers of the lenses the same distance apart as the centers of the wearer's pupils. If prism was prescribed, the point on each lens where the prism amount is exactly correct should be the same distance apart as the centers of the wearer's pupils. The distance between the wearer's pupils is called the *pupillary distance*, or *PD*. (For a discussion of how to measure the wearer's PD, refer to a good dispensing book such as Brooks and Borish, *System for Ophthalmic Dispensing*.) We call the distance between the geometrical centers of the lenses in a pair of glasses the *frame PD*, or *FPD*. This is 1/2 of the right lens A, plus the DBL, plus 1/2 of the left lens A. Since the right and left lens A measurements are usually equal, the FPD = A + DBL.

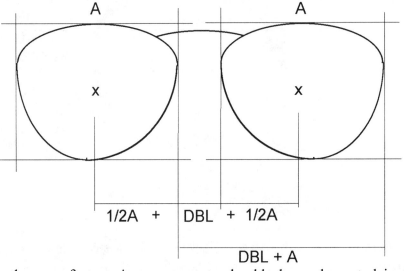

Although the manufacturers' measurements should always be noted in the wearer's records, for the laboratory calculations measure the frame using the boxing system instead of using the manufacturers' marked measurements.

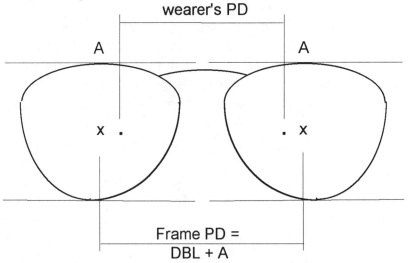

x is the geometric center of each lens.
· is the desired optical center of each lens.

Compare the wearer's PD and the frame PD. If the optical centers are centered in the frame, the glasses PD will be equal to the frame PD. If we take one-half of the difference between the wearer's PD and the frame PD, and offset the optical centers by this amount in each lens, then the completed glasses PD will be equal to the wearer's PD. This process is called *decentering the lens,* because we are moving the optical center away from the geometrical center of the lens.

$$\boxed{\text{DECENTRATION} = 1/2(\text{FPD} - \text{PD})}$$

where PD is binocular.

If the wearer's eyes are not symmetrical, or if you are preparing progressive bifocal lenses, you may be given *monocular PDs.* Monocular PDs are the distance from the center of the wearer's nose to the center of the pupil of each eye. In this case, divide the FPD in half, and subtract each of the two monocular PDs.

$$\boxed{\begin{array}{l} \text{OD DECENTRATION} = 1/2\ \text{FPD} - \text{PD}_{OD}, \\ \quad \text{where } \text{PD}_{OD} \text{ is monocular.} \\ \text{OS DECENTRATION} = 1/2\ \text{FPD} - \text{PD}_{OS}, \\ \quad \text{where } \text{PD}_{OS} \text{ is monocular.} \end{array}}$$

The *pattern difference,* or *P measurement*, is A − B. P is an indication of how similar the A and B measurements are. For example, P = 0 for a round frame.

EXAMPLE: On the following diagram, determine:
  a. the A, B, DBL, PFD, and P using the boxing system.
  b. the D and DBL using the datum system.
  c. the decentration needed if the wearer's PD is 58mm.
  d. the decentration needed if the wearer's monocular PD is 28/30.

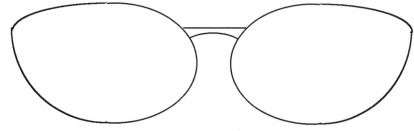

Eyewires made of very thin metal.

Begin by drawing rectangles around each lens, and measure 1/2 of the A and 1/2 of the B to locate the geometrical center. Measure both lenses. They will not always be the same.

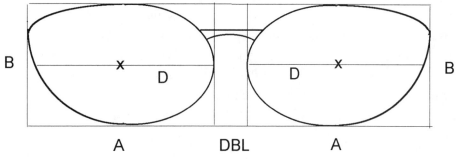

a. A = 51mm
    B = 32mm
    DBL = 9mm
    FPD = 60mm
    P = 19mm

b. D = 49mm
    DBL = 9mm

c. FPD – PD = 60 – 58 = 2. 1/2 of 2 is 1 mm decentration in OU.
d. 1/2 of 60 is 30. OD decentration is 30 – 28 = 2 mm in.
    OS decentration is 30 – 30 = 0 mm in.

EFFECTIVE DIAMETER

The *effective diameter* of a lens, or the ED of the lens, is defined as two times the longest radius of the lens. Once the geometrical center of the lens has been identified, find the point on the eyewire that is the farthest from the center, measure the distance, and multiply by two. The longest measurement may be to any of the corners of the frame. The longest measurement on the frame from eyewire to eyewire is **not** the ED.

EXAMPLE: On the frame on the last example, the longest radius is 26.5 mm, so the ED is 53mm. The longest distance from eyewire to eyewire is only 51mm.

SEGMENT HEIGHT AND DROP

On a bifocal lens, we need to know where the center of the top of the segment will be with respect to the geometrical center of the lens. The center of the top of the segment is sometimes called the *bifocal reference point*.

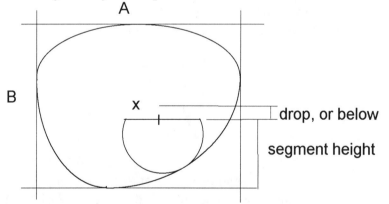

x is the geometrical center of the lens.

The *segment height* is the distance from the top of the bifocal segment to the lowest point of the edge of the lens. The point on the lens edge that is directly below the segment is not always the lowest point, as can be seen from the diagram above. The *segment drop* or *below* is 1/2 B – seg height. In the diagram above, B = 43, seg height = 18, and drop = 43/2 – 18 = 21.5 – 18 = 3.5mm. Note that for progressive addition lenses, the segment height is to the fitting cross, and will usually be *above* rather than *below*. When measuring the desired segment height for a plastic frame, add 1/2mm to the segment height for the lower bevel of the lens.

FRAME MEASUREMENT EXERCISES

On each of the following diagrams determine:

    a. the A, B, DBL, FPD, ED, and P using the boxing system.

    b. the D and DBL using the datum system.

    c. the segment height and below or above.

    d. the distance decentration needed if the wearer's distance PD is 61mm.

    e. the distance decentration needed if the wearer's distance monocular PD is 29/32.

1. Thin metal

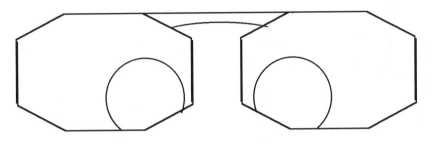

(Use the top of the round segment for the segment height.)

2. semi-rimless, nylon suspension

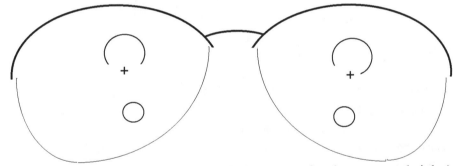

(Use the +, which is the fitting cross, for the segment height.)

3. Thick zyl

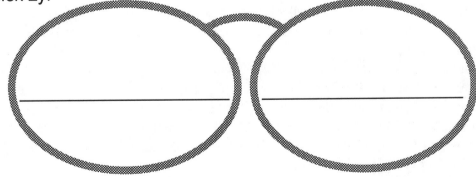

MINIMUM BLANK SIZE

We use the ***minimum blank size*** when cutting out single vision lenses to help us determine if the lens needs to be surfaced, or if it can be cut from a stock lens.

If there is no decentration of the optical center (for a plano lens, for example), the minimum blank size will be equal to the ED of the frame. If the lens must be decentered by one millimeter, then we need 1mm in *each direction* on the lens, so we would add 2mm to the ED. Similarly, if the decentration is 3mm, then we need 3mm in both directions, or 6mm plus the ED.

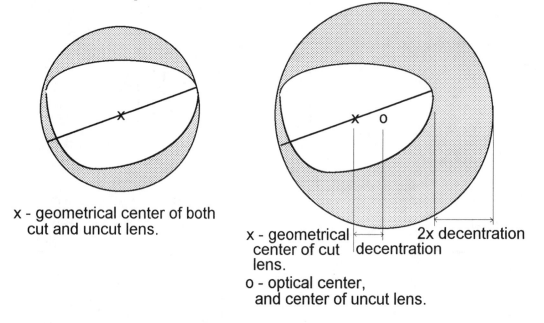

x - geometrical center of both cut and uncut lens.

x - geometrical center of cut lens.

o - optical center, and center of uncut lens.

Since the lens moved by the amount of decentration, the *radius* of the necessary uncut lens increased by the amount of decentration, and the *diameter* increased by twice the amount of decentration. The very edge of the lens blank may have a nick or a mold seam, so for practical purposes some people add 1-2mm to the amount needed for the minimum blank size. Thus,

> minimum blank size = ED + (2)(decentration) + 2mm.

Depending on the shape of the lens, the direction of the ED, and the condition of the edge, the lens may cut out of a smaller blank. The formula gives a "safe cutout" measurement, which is the largest size that the blank will need to be for a lens with a given decentration and ED.

Minimum blank size for a multifocal depends on the segment drop, the placement of the distance optical center with respect to the segment, the decentration, and the ED. Use a chart supplied by the lens manufacturer if one is available. Of particular interest are the charts supplied by most progressive addition lens manufacturers. A discussion about making your own minimum blank size chart for multifocals may be found in Brooks, *Understanding Lens Surfacing*, pages 25-29.

EXAMPLES: What is the minimum blank size for a frame with ED of 55 and FPD of 65 if the wearer's PD is 62? What is the minimum blank size for the same frame if the wearer's PD is 53?

> If the wearer's PD is 62, then the total decentration is 65 − 62 = 3mm. For one lens we use 1/2 of the total decentration; for minimum blank size we multiply by 2 again. So we can just use the difference as is. The minimum blank size is ED + twice the decentration + 2mm = 55 + 3 + 2 = 60mm. The lens will cut out of a stock lens blank that has a 60mm diameter or more.

> For the person with a 53mm PD, 65 − 53 = 12, and the minimum blank size is 55 + 12 + 2 = 69mm.

MINIMUM BLANK SIZE EXERCISES

1. What is the minimum blank size for a wearer PD of 60, if the A = 52, B = 48, DBL = 18, and ED = 55?

2. Compute the minimum blank size if the frame PD is 61, A = 51, P = 2, and ED = 51, if the requested final PD is 58.

3. A frame has measurements of A = 59, B = 50, DBL = 18, ED = 63, and a requested PD of 35/37 (monocular distance). What is the minimum blank size for this pair of glasses?

BASE CURVES

There are several definitions of a base curve.

> 1. *The **base curve of a lens** is the curve on the lens from which all of the other curves will be computed.* On a spherical single vision lens, the base curve is usually the curve on the front or convex side. On a toric single vision lens, the base curve is the curve on the spherical surface, which is on the front or convex side if the lens is made in minus cylinder form.
> 2. *The **base curve of a multifocal lens** is the curve on the surface containing the segment.* This surface will be spherical for any bifocal lens where the segment is molded on the surface. On a fused glass bifocal lens, the surface with the segment can be given a toric surface, but it usually is not.
> 3. *The **base curve of a toric surface** is the flattest curve on the surface.* In a lens that has been ground in minus cylinder form, this is the flattest curve on the concave surface. In a lens that has been ground in plus cylinder form, this is the flattest or least steep curve on the convex surface.

Definitions number one and two are the definitions that are used to choose a base curve for a prescription. Definition number three will be used in the discussion of toric transposition.

BASE CURVE SELECTION

Before corrected curve series lenses were developed, base curves were chosen to keep the ocular surface as close to −6.00D as possible. In plus lenses, this can be done by adding +6.00D to the spherical equivalent of the lens power. In minus lenses, the rule of thumb is to add 1/2 of the (negative) spherical equivalent to +6.00D. This rule of thumb is called *Vogel's Rule*. For example, if the Rx is +3.50, the base curve could be (+6.00) + (+3.50) = +9.50. But if the Rx is −3.50, then the base curve is (+6.00) + (−3.50/2) = (+6.00) + (−1.75) = +4.25. (Note: The spherical equivalent of a spherical power *is* the sphere.)

Corrected curve design lenses were developed to minimize lens aberrations called *marginal astigmatism* (also called *oblique astigmatism*) and *curvature of field*. The corrected curve series typically have base curves such as +2.25D or +7.25D. When you look up a lens power on a chart to determine what base curve to use, you are probably making a corrected curve lens. For any particular prescription, the base curve that will minimize or eliminate marginal astigmatism is not the exact same curve that will minimize or eliminate curvature of field aberration. Also, using the best base curve for every prescription would result in having to stock a very large variety of base curves. Every lens manufacturer's corrected curve series is the result of making compromises between minimizing the two aberrations and the need to control inventory; therefore, different corrected curve lens series may recommend different (but similar) base curves for any particular prescription.

Some base curve charts require that we transpose to minus cylinder form and then look up the prescription on a table to find the recommended base curve. Others require that we determine the spherical equivalent of the prescription and determine where it falls in a grouping of prescriptions such as the following:

Sample chart for CR39:

BASE CURVE SELECTION CHART*	
Sph. Equiv.	Base Curve
+8.50 to +12.50**	+12.25D
+5.50 to +8.25	+10.25D
+1.50 to +5.25	+8.25D
−1.25 to +1.25	+6.25D
−1.50 to −5.25	+4.25D
−5.50 to −9.25	+2.25D
−9.50 and above	+0.25D
** Aspheric curves recommended.	

EXAMPLES:

1. An Rx of −5.00D would be placed on a +3.50 base curve using Vogel's rule. Using the Base Curve Selection Chart above, the Rx of −5.00D would be ground on a +4.25D base curve.

*Not an official corrected curve chart.

2. An Rx of +4.50 +1.00 x090 would be placed on a +11.00D base curve using Vogel's rule. Using the Base Curve Selection Chart above, this Rx would be ground on a +8.25D base curve.

Notes:
1. Vogel's rule gives a "place to start" when you are taking a multiple choice examination. Use it to find an approximate base curve, and then choose the answer that is either the closest or the next flatter.
2. When a base curve is specified on an order or on the Rx, ANSI standards state that the base curve supplied may be within ±0.75D of the curve requested.
3. When specifying base curve, most authorities recommend
    a. that new lenses be placed on the same base curve as the old lens base curve *if reasonable*;
    b. that both lenses in a pair of glasses be on the same base curve *if reasonable* (use the base curve recommended for the strongest lens);
    c. that high plus prescriptions be placed on aspheric base curves;
    d. that the base curve for a plus lens be flattened slightly for insertion in difficult frames.
4. Many wholesale labs stock one or two base curve series and may not be able to grind the prescription on exactly the same base curve requested. Rejecting a base curve that is within ±0.75D of the curve requested may result in delays in delivery and an increased charge.

BASE CURVE SELECTION EXERCISES

1. What base curve does Vogel's Rule call for if the Rx is −3.00 −2.00 x180? What base curve does the selection chart on the previous page call for?

2. What base curve does the chart indicate for a lens of power +3.00 −2.50 x090? What does Vogel's Rule call for?

3. What base curve might be used for a −6.00DS lens using Vogel's rule? Using the chart?

TORIC TRANSPOSITION

The purpose of *toric transposition* is to show what curves will be ground on the surfaces of the lens. The steps in toric transposition are:
1. Place the base curve on the diagram of the lens. If the Rx is to be made in minus cylinder form, then the base curve will have plus power and will be on the convex surface. If the Rx is to be made in plus cylinder form, then the base curve will have minus power and will be on the concave surface. If the written prescription is not in the correct cylinder form, transpose it first.
2. Compute the flattest curve on the second surface of the lens. If the Rx is in the correct cylinder form, this is the curve needed to give the spherical power of the prescription

using the nominal power formula on page 33. This curve is the toric surface base curve. (See number 3 of the definitions of base curve on page 113.)

3. Compute the power curve on the toric surface of the lens. This is the curve found in step 2, plus the amount of the prescribed cylinder.

EXAMPLE: Using a base curve of +4.25D, show the surface curves of a lens having the Rx −3.00 −1.00 x090.

1. The base curve of the lens is to be +4.25, on the convex side of the lens. (If the Rx had not been in minus cylinder form we would flat transpose it.)

$$+4.25D$$
$$========$$

2. To get a sphere power of −3.00D using a base curve of +4.25D, we need a toric base curve of −7.25D. $[D_2 = D_N − D_1 = −3.00 −(+4.25) = −7.25D]$

$$+4.25D$$
$$========$$
$$−7.25D$$

3. For the power curve add the amount of the cylinder to the toric base curve.

$$(−7.25) + (−1.00) = −8.25$$
$$+4.25D$$
$$========$$
$$−7.25 \circleddash −8.25$$

Note: Toric transposition sometimes shows the axis for the toric base curve and for the power curve. Thus the toric surface in this example could be written either −7.25 x090 $\circleddash$ −8.25 x180 (power/axis) *or* −7.25 x180 $\circleddash$ −8.25 x090 (crossed cylinder notation) depending on the equipment used in the laboratory.

TORIC TRANSPOSITION EXERCISES

1. Given the Rx −2.00 −1.50 x045 and the base curve +4.25D, what are the surface curves?

2. Given the base curve of −6.00 and the Rx pl + 0.50 x180, what are the surface curves? (Note: The Rx is to be ground in plus cylinder form.)

3. Show the toric transposition of the Rx +5.00 +1.50 x060, using a base curve of +10.25D.

4. What is the toric transposition for the Rx −8.50 −1.25 x115, with a base curve of +2.00D?

TRUE POWER FORMULA

In Section II, when we discussed the surface power formula, we learned that the power of a surface depends on the radius of curvature of the surface and the index of refraction of the material of the surface. The lens clock, the surfacing laps in most ophthalmic labs, and most generator calibrations are based on making or measuring curves on a material of index of refraction 1.530. For low power Rx's in crown glass, index 1.523, it is acceptable to use tools with index 1.530. We may correct for the index when using CR39 or high index materials . The formula used to convert the power *marked* on the tool to the actual (or *true*) power created by the tool is:

$$\frac{D_{MARKED}}{D_{TRUE}} = \frac{0.53}{n_{TRUE} - 1}$$

where D_{MARKED} = the power marked on the lap or the lens clock reading,

D_{TRUE} = the actual power of the surface,

n_{TRUE} = the index of refraction of the lens material.

The tool needed (D_{MARKED}) to grind the curve that will have the actual power (D_{TRUE}) is

$$D_{MARKED} = \frac{0.53}{n_{TRUE} - 1} \times D_{TRUE}$$

Or, the true power of a surface (D_{TRUE}) that clocks at (D_{MARKED}) is

$$D_{TRUE} = \frac{n_{TRUE} - 1}{0.53} \times D_{MARKED}$$

EXAMPLE 1: What tool would be used to grind an actual (or true) power of −5.00D on a lens made of CR39?

$$D_{MARKED} = \frac{0.53}{n_{TRUE} - 1} \times D_{TRUE}$$

$$D_{MARKED} = \frac{0.53}{1.498 - 1} \times -5.00 = \frac{0.53}{0.498} \times -5.00 = -5.32$$

Corrected to the next highest 1/8D, the tool used would be −5.37D.

EXAMPLE 2: What is the actual (or true) surface power of a polycarbonate surface, n = 1.586, if the lens clock shows +7.25D?

$$D_{TRUE} = \frac{n_{TRUE} - 1}{0.53} \times D_{MARKED}$$

$$D_{TRUE} = \frac{1.586 - 1}{0.53} \times +7.25 = \frac{0.586}{0.53} \times +7.25 = +8.01$$

Although the lens clock will read +7.25D on this surface, it actually has a power of +8.01 because it is made out of polycarbonate.

We do not change TRUE power to one-eighth diopter steps because we are not going to make the lens using a tool, nor are we going to measure it with a lens clock. We change MARKED power to one-eighth diopter steps because the marked power results in an actual tool which will be used. In some labs, MARKED powers are automatically changed to the next highest one-eighth diopter step; in the exercises below, change to the nearest one-eighth diopter.

TRUE POWER EXERCISES

(Change marked power to 1/8 diopter steps. Round true power to two decimal places.)

1. If the lens clock reads −3.25D on a material with an index of 1.586 (polycarbonate), what is the true (or actual) power of the curve?

2. If the lens clock reads +10.75D on a material with index of refraction of 1.498, what is the true (or actual) power of the surface?

3. If we want an actual (or true) power of −7.50D on a surface made of a material with index of 1.60, what tool would we use?

4. If we want an actual power of −3.75 on a surface made of CR39 (n = 1.498), what tool would be used?

5. You are to make a lens with an Rx of −8.50 −2.00 x090 of a high index plastic having an index of refraction of 1.66. The base curve chosen for this lens reads +1.25 on the lens clock. What tool will be used to make the back surface? STEPS:
   a. What is the true power of the base curve marked +1.25, made of a material with index of refraction of 1.66?

   b. Toric transpose for the actual powers needed on the back of the lens.

   c. Convert each of the back powers to marked powers. The result is what the tool will be, and what the lens clock will show, when the lens is finished. Since you will choose tools with this power, change to the nearest 1/8D.

THINK ABOUT IT: Using the curves found in 5.c, compute the power that the lens would have had if the lens were made of a material with index 1.530. Why is it difficult to estimate the power of a high index lens just by using the readings from the lens clock?

SAGITTAL DEPTH AND LENS THICKNESS

The term *sag* refers to the *sagittal depth* of a curve or surface. If a straight edge is placed across the surface at a particular diameter, the sagittal depth is the farthest distance that the surface is from the straight edge.

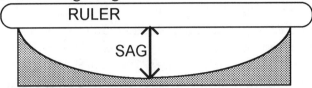

The formula for the sagittal depth of a surface is

$$SAG = r - \sqrt{r^2 - (d/2)^2}$$

where   d is the diameter of the surface, in mm

           r is the radius of curvature of the surface, in mm

(d is the distance between the two points where the ruler touches the surface.)

Note: The measurements may be in any unit, as long as r, d, and sag are *all the same unit*.

Remember from Section III, pages 35-36, that r, the radius of curvature, is equal to (n–1)/D. This formula may be rewritten as

$$SAG = \frac{n-1}{D} - \sqrt{\left(\frac{n-1}{D}\right)^2 - \left(\frac{d}{2}\right)^2}$$

EXAMPLE 1: A surface made of polycarbonate has a true power of –6.00D and a diameter of 60mm. What is the sag of the surface?

    n = 1.586,

    r = (n–1)/D = (1.586–1)/(6) = 0.0977m = 97.7mm.

    d/2 = 60/2 = 30

$$SAG = r - \sqrt{r^2 - [d/2]^2}$$

$$SAG = 97.7 - \sqrt{97.7^2 - 30^2} = 97.7 - \sqrt{9545.29 - 900}$$

$$= 97.7 - \sqrt{8645.29} = 97.7 - 93.0 = 4.7mm$$

Notice that the sign of the radius of curvature (actually the sign of the surface power) is not used in this form of the sagittal depth formula. In Section VII we will deal with the sign of r. We will adjust for not using the sign of r here when combining the sagittal depths of the two surfaces of the lens.

The sag of a flat or plano surface is 0. Using the sag of the –6.00 surface made of polycarbonate, the edge thickness of a plano-concave lens with power –6.00 can now be found.

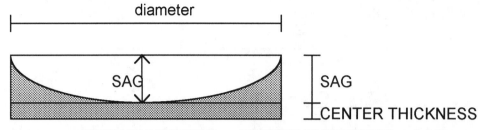

diameter

SAG

SAG
CENTER THICKNESS

EDGE THICKNESS = CENTER THICKNESS + SAG

If a center thickness of 1.5mm is requested, the edge thickness of the 60mm diameter lens will be 4.7mm + 1.5mm = **6.2mm**.

EXAMPLE 2: If the –6.00D lens is made with a base curve of +3.00D, a back curve of –9.00D, a diameter of 60mm, and a center thickness of 1.5mm, what is the edge thickness? (These curves are true values, not marked values.)

$r = (n – 1) / D$

$r_{FRONT} = (1.586 – 1)/3 = 0.1953m =$ **195mm**

$r_{BACK} = (1.586 – 1)/9 = 0.0651m =$ **65mm**

$$SAG = r - \sqrt{r^2 - [d/2]^2}$$

$$SAG_{front} = 195 - \sqrt{195^2 - 30^2} = 195 - \sqrt{38025 - 900}$$
$$= 195 - \sqrt{37125} = 195 - 192.68 = 2.3mm$$

$$SAG_{back} = 65 - \sqrt{65^2 - 30^2} = 65 - \sqrt{4225 - 900}$$
$$= 65 - \sqrt{3325} = 65 - 57.66 = 7.3mm$$

-9.00D

+3.00D

sag of -9.00 = 7.3mm
sag of +3.00 = 2.3mm
difference between sags is 5.0mm
(assuming 0 center thickness)

The difference between the two sags is 5.0mm, which is thicker than the plano/convex form of the lens. Adding the requested center thickness of 1.5mm results in an edge thickness of **6.5mm**.

Edge thickness of lens =

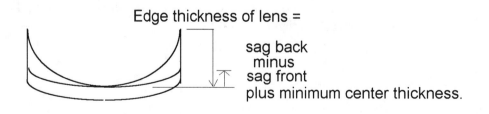

sag back
minus
sag front
plus minimum center thickness.

The formula for the *edge thickness of a minus lens* is

> **EDGE THICKNESS =**
> $SAG_{BACK} - SAG_{FRONT} + CENTER\ THICKNESS$

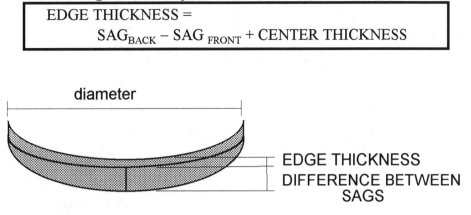

diameter

EDGE THICKNESS
DIFFERENCE BETWEEN
SAGS

The *center thickness of a plus lens* is

> **CENTER THICKNESS =**
> $SAG_{FRONT} - SAG_{BACK} + EDGE\ THICKNESS$

EXAMPLE 3: What is the center thickness of a +6.00D lens, n = 1.530, if the edge thickness is 2.00mm, the lens diameter is 60mm, and the base curve is = +10.00D?

$r = (n-1) / D$

$r_{FRONT} = (1.530 - 1)/10 = 0.053m = \textbf{53mm}$

$r_{BACK} = (1.530 - 1)/4 = 0.1325m = \textbf{133mm}$

$SAG = r - \sqrt{r^2 - [d/2]^2}$

$$SAG_{front} = 53 - \sqrt{53^2 - 30^2} = 53 - \sqrt{2809 - 900}$$
$$= 53 - \sqrt{1909} = 53 - 43.7 = 9.3mm$$

$$SAG_{back} = 133 - \sqrt{133^2 - 30^2} = 133 - \sqrt{17689 - 900}$$
$$= 133 - \sqrt{16789} = 133 - 129.57 = 3.4mm$$

CENTER THICKNESS = DIFF. between SAGs + EDGE THICKNESS
= (9.3 − 3.4) + 2.0 = 5.9 + 2.0 = **7.9mm**

EXAMPLE 4: What is the approximate edge thickness of a −6.00D polycarbonate lens, n = 1.586, if the center thickness is 1.5 mm, the base curve is a true +2.00D, and the lens diameter is 60mm?

$r = (n-1) / D$

$r_{FRONT} = (1.586 - 1)/2 = 0.293m = \textbf{293mm}$

$r_{BACK} = (1.586 - 1)/8 = 0.07325m = \textbf{73mm}$

$$\text{SAG} = r - \sqrt{r^2 - [d/2]^2}$$

$$\text{SAG}_{front} = 293 - \sqrt{293^2 - 30^2} = 293 - \sqrt{85849 - 900}$$

$$= 293 - \sqrt{84949} = 293 - 291.46 = 1.5\text{mm}$$

$$\text{SAG}_{back} = 73 - \sqrt{73^2 - 30^2} = 73 - \sqrt{5329 - 900}$$

$$= 73 - \sqrt{4429} = 73 - 66.55 = 6.4\text{mm}$$

EDGE THICKNESS = DIFF between SAGs + CENTER THICKNESS

$$= (6.4 - 1.5) + 1.5 = 4.9 + 1.5 = \textbf{6.4mm}$$

APPROXIMATE SAG FORMULA

The following *approximate* sag of a lens is in general use, and for low power lenses gives an acceptable approximation for the lens thickness.

$$\boxed{\text{SAG} = \frac{(d/2)^2\, D}{2000(n-1)}}$$

where   d is the diameter of the surface in mm,
D is the lens power,
n is the index of refraction for the material from which the lens is made.

EXAMPLE 5: What is the approximate center thickness of a +6.00D plastic lens, n = 1.530, if the edge thickness is 2.0 mm and the lens diameter is 60mm?

CENTER THICKNESS = SAG + EDGE THICKNESS

$$\text{SAG} = \frac{(d/2)^2\, D}{2000(n-1)}$$

$$\text{SAG} = \frac{(30)^2\, 6.00}{2000(0.523)} = \frac{5400}{1046} = 5.2\text{mm}$$

CENTER THICKNESS = 5.2mm + 2.0mm = 7.2mm

In example 3, the exact formula gave us 7.9mm for this sag.

EXAMPLE 6: What is the approximate edge thickness of a −6.00D polycarbonate lens, n = 1.586, if the center thickness is 1.5 mm and the lens diameter is 60mm?

EDGE THICKNESS = SAG + CENTER THICKNESS

$$\text{SAG} = \frac{(d/2)^2\, D}{2000(n-1)}$$

$$SAG = \frac{(30)^2 \, 6.00}{2000(0.586)} = 4.6mm$$

THICKNESS = 4.6mm + 1.5mm = 6.1 mm

In example 4, the exact formula gave us 6.4mm for this thickness.

SAG FORMULA AND LENS THICKNESS EXERCISES
(Round radius of curvature to mm and sag to tenths of mm.)

1. What is the approximate center thickness of a +2.50D lens with n = 1.498 if the edge thickness is to be 2.0mm at a diameter of 56mm? Use the approximation formula.

2. Redo the calculations from problem 1.
   a. Choose a base curve from the table on page 114.
   b. Use the true power formula to convert to true power; then find the true back curve.
   c. Use these two true power curves to find the actual sags of the curves.
   d. Find the approximate center thickness of the +2.50D lens.

PRISM THICKNESS

The base thickness t of a prismatic lens with no power may be found using the formula

$$t = \frac{d\,P}{100(n-1)} \quad \text{or} \quad P = \frac{t\,(100[n-1])}{d}$$

where P = prism power,
   t = thickness in mm,
   d = diameter of the lens in mm.

This formula assumes that the apex of the prism is 0mm or knife-edge.

EXAMPLE: You are given a prescription of pl, 5^ΔBO OU. The wearer chooses a frame of 50 □ 18. The finished lens will have a minimum edge thickness of 2.0mm. What will the maximum edge thickness be?

Since this Rx has no power, we do not need to be concerned with decentration. Since the prism is base out, which is horizontal, the diameter of the lens needed is the A size of the frame, 50mm. If the lenses are made of plastic, n=1.50, then the base thickness is

$$t = \frac{d\,P}{100(n-1)} = \frac{(50)(5)}{(100)(0.5)} = \frac{250}{50} = 5mm$$

Adding a minimum edge thickness of 2.0mm to the 5mm will give a thickness of **7.0mm** on the outside edge of each lens.

Notice that the thickness of the base is equal to the prism power for a lens of diameter 50mm and a material of index 1.50. The general rule of thumb for prism thickness is:

> For a 50mm diameter lens made of material of n = 1.50, the difference between thicknesses of the base and the apex of the prism in mm will equal the amount of the prism power in diopters.

If the material is high index, the prism base thickness will be less than the amount of the prism. (Why?) If the lens is bigger than 50mm, the prism base thickness will be more than the amount of the prism. If the lens is smaller than 50mm, the prism base thickness will be less than the amount of the prism. Why?

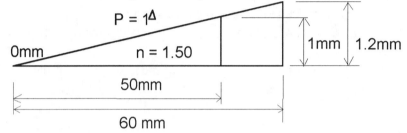

Maximum edge thickness for a prismatic lens with plano power is the sum of the prism base thickness plus the minimum edge thickness for the ED of the lens.

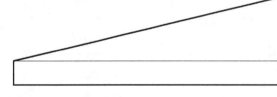

Maximum edge thickness for a prismatic lens with plus power is also the sum of the prism base thickness plus the minimum edge thickness for the minimum blank size of the lens. Center thickness for a prismatic lens with plus power is the sum of the sag of the lens, the minimum edge thickness, and one-half of the prism base thickness.

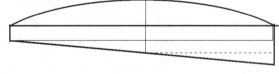

> For a plus lens,
> THICKEST EDGE = PRISM BASE THICKNESS + MINIMUM EDGE THICKNESS
> CENTER THICKNESS = SAG + MINIMUM EDGE THICKNESS + 1/2 PRISM BASE THICKNESS

On minus power prismatic lenses, adding the edge thickness, the minimum center thickness, and the prism base gives more thickness than necessary, since it results in an optical center thickness that is thicker than necessary. Using 1/2 of the prism base thickness amount (or finding the thickness of the prism portion at one-half the ED) will give an amount which may be added to the sum of the Rx sag and minimum center thickness for the thickest edge amount.

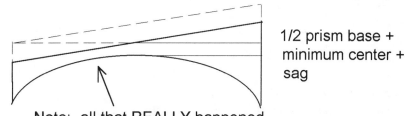

1/2 prism base +
minimum center +
sag

Note: all that REALLY happened
is the optical center moved!

> For a minus lens,
> THICKEST EDGE = 1/2 PRISM BASE THICKNESS +
> MINIMUM CENTER THICKNESS + SAG

Can you identify the new optical center on the plus prismatic lens on page 124?

EXAMPLE: 1. What are the approximate maximum edge and center thicknesses for the Rx +4.00DS 2$^\Delta$BU for a polycarbonate (n = 1.586) lens with a minimum blank size of 48, a sag of 2.1mm, and a minimum thickness of 1.5mm?

Step 1. Determine the prism base thickness.

$$ t = \frac{d\,P}{100(n-1)} = \frac{(48)(2)}{(100)(0.586)} = \frac{96}{58.6} = 1.6mm $$

Step 2. Determine thickest edge.
Thickest edge = minimum thickness + prism base thickness = 1.5 + 1.6 = **3.1mm**

Step 3. Determine center thickness.
Center thickness = minimum thickness + sag + 1/2 prism base
= 1.5 + 2.1 + 1/2(1.6) = **4.4mm**

Note: The thickness is a maximum and an approximation. Since the prism is BU, some of the thickest edge will be cut off.

EXAMPLE 2. What is the approximate maximum edge thickness for Rx −3.00DS 2$^\Delta$BI for a CR39 lens with a minimum blank size of 54mm, a sag of 2.4mm, and a minimum center thickness of 2.2mm? Redo it, using a plastic with an index of refraction of 1.66, and a sag of 1.9mm.

Using CR39:
Step 1. Determine the prism base thickness.

$$t = \frac{d\ P}{100(n-1)} = \frac{(54)(2)}{(100)(0.498)} = \frac{108}{49.8} = \textbf{2.2mm}$$

Step 2. Determine thickest edge.
Thickest edge using CR39 = minimum thickness + sag + 1/2 prism base thickness

$$= 2.2 + 2.4 + (2.2/2) = \textbf{5.7mm}$$

Using n = 1.66:
Step 1. Determine the prism base thickness.

$$t = \frac{d\ P}{100(n-1)} = \frac{(54)(2)}{(100)(0.66)} = \frac{108}{66} = \textbf{1.6mm}$$

Step 2. Determine thickest edge.
Thickest edge using high index = 2.2 + 1.9 + (1.6/2) = **4.9mm**

Again, note that after edging the lens to fit the frame some of this thickness will have been removed.

THICKNESS EXERCISES
(Round to tenths of mm.)

1. What are the approximate maximum edge and center thicknesses for the Rx +5.50DS, 3$^\Delta$BO, for a polycarbonate (n = 1.586) lens with a minimum blank size of 44mm, a sag of 2.4mm, and a minimum thickness of 1.5mm?

2. What are the center thickness and maximum edge thickness for the same lens in question 1 using CR39 (n = 1.498), sag of 2.9mm and minimum edge of 2.0mm?

SECTION VI: ADVANCED LENS FORMULAS

MARTIN'S FORMULA FOR LENS TILT

The position of a lens in front of the eye changes the effect of the lens on the eye system. One example is vertex distance change. Pantoscopic tilt and face form will also change the effective power of the lens. Changing the tilt of the lens induces *marginal astigmatism*, also called *oblique astigmatism*, a lens aberration.

Pantoscopic tilt changes the effective sphere power of the lens and induces cylinder power on the 180 meridian. For a plus sphere lens, plus cylinder is induced. For a minus sphere lens, minus cylinder is induced. Face form will change the sphere power of the lens and induce cylinder power on the 90 meridian. For small amounts of tilt, the formula for the new effective power of the lens is:

$$S' = S[1+(\sin\alpha)^2/2n]$$
$$C' = S'(\tan\alpha)^2$$

where S' = the new spherical power,

S = original sphere power,

α = the degrees of tilt,

n = index of refraction of the lens material,

C' = the induced cylinder on the axis of rotation.

EXAMPLE 1: A +10.00D lens made of CR39 ($n = 1.498$) is tilted 15°. What is the effective power for this lens?

$$S' = S[1+(\sin\alpha)^2] = (+10.00)(1+[\sin 15]^2/2[1.498])$$
$$= (10)(1+0.06699/2.996) = (+10.00)(1.02235) = \textbf{+10.22D}$$
$$C' = S'(\tan\alpha) = (+10.22)(\tan 15)^2 = (+10.22)(0.0718) = \textbf{+0.73 x180}$$

Effective Rx +10.22 +0.73 x180

The answers are not changed to 1/8D because this effective power is not going to be ordered from a lab or recorded in the wearer's records.

This formula assumes that the optical center of the lens is directly in front of the wearer's pupil. The effect of pantoscopic tilt on the prescription can be changed by changing the position of the optical center. To eliminate unwanted power changes and eliminate marginal astigmatism, the general rule is

Lower the optical center 1mm for
every 2 degrees of pantoscopic tilt.

Note: You may have seen the new sphere formula in the form $S' = S[1+(\sin\alpha)^2/3]$. This formula works for CR39 and for crown glass, and is a very close approximation for high index materials.

EXAMPLE 2: What is the effective Rx if the following glasses are fitted with the OC in front of the pupil and with 10 degrees of pantoscopic tilt? The glasses are made of polycarbonate, n = 1.586.

Rx: OD –8.50DS

OS –9.25DS

OD $S' = S[1+(\sin \alpha)^2] = (-8.50)(1 + (\sin10)^2/2(1.586)$
$= (-8.50)(1 + (0.030)/(3.172) = (-8.50)(1.0095)$

$S' = -8.58D$

$C' = S'(\tan \alpha) = (-8.58)(\tan10)^2 = (-8.58)(0.031) = -0.27D$

OS $S' = S[1+(\sin \alpha)^2] = (-9.25)(1 + (\sin10)^2/2(1.586)$
$= (-9.25)(1 + (0.030)/(3.172) = (-9.25)(1.0095)$

$S' = -9.34D$

$C' = S'(\tan \alpha) = (-9.34)(\tan10)^2 = (-9.34)(0.031) = -0.29D$

Effective Rx OD –8.58 –0.27 x180

OS –9.34 –0.29 x180

EXAMPLE 3: What is the effective Rx for the following Rx if the glasses have 15 degrees of face form, and the pd is made normally? The glasses are made of 1.66 plastic.

Rx +7.00 –2.00 x180 OU

The prescription already has some cylinder in it. Since the tilt will induce cylinder on the 90th meridian, first transpose the problem to the 90th meridian, then use the sphere power in the exercise.

Rx +5.00 +2.00 x090

$S' = S[1+(\sin \alpha)^2] = (+5.00)(1 + (\sin15)^2/2(1.66)$
$= (+5.00)(1 + (0.067)/(3.32) = (+5.00)(1.020)$

$S' = +5.10D$

$C' = S'(\tan \alpha) = (+5.10)(\tan15)^2 = (+5.10)(0.072) = +0.37 \ x090$

C' is added to the old cylinder power, since they are at the same axis. The new cylinder power is +2.00 +0.37 = **+2.37D**

The effective Rx is +5.10 +2.37 x090 or +7.47 – 2.37 x180.

Note: *Compensating the Rx for tilt, increasing the pd 1mm for every 2 degrees of face form, and using retroscopic tilt to correct for an oc which is above the pupil, are NOT recommended procedures.*

What if the prescription had cylinder with an axis other than 90 or 180? The result of the cylinder and axis calculations will be obliquely crossed cylinders, and involves the use of both Martin's formula and Thompson's formula, on pages 135-137. Calculation of the sphere power, however, is beyond the scope of this document. Note that if the cylinder is small with respect to the sphere power, an approximation may be calculated using just the sphere of the prescription.

In the following exercises notice that low pantoscopic tilt or a small amount of face form introduce very little error.

MARTINS FORMULA FOR TILT EXERCISES
(Round answers to hundredths of a diopter.)

1. If a –6.00D polycarbonate (n = 1.586) sphere is tilted pantoscopically 20 degrees, what is the effective sphere power and the amount of cylinder induced at the optical center?

2. If a +10.00D sphere made of n=1.66 plastic is tilted pantoscopically 5 degrees, what is the effective Rx at the optical center?

3. Given a +4.50 polycarbonate (n = 1.586) lens with 20 degrees of positive face form because the wearer insists it gives him side protection when riding on his bike, what is the effective lens power?

SPECTACLE MAGNIFICATION

Plus lenses are often considered to be magnifiers. A hyperope wears a plus lens because this lens adds just enough power to the eye system to bring the focal plane to the retina, not because it magnifies the image. A presbyope wears extra plus power (or less minus power) because that is what is needed to bring the image of a close object to a focus on the retina. *Magnification* induced by the glasses lens or the contact lens *is a side effect* of the lens power.

The amount of magnification that any particular lens will add to the eye system depends on a variety of factors. The factors are:
1. the thickness of the lens,
2. the material used to make the lens,
3. the distance the lens is from the eye, and
4. the curvature of the front surface of the lens.

These factors all have to work together to give the correct focal length. For any particular prescription, there are many different combinations of these factors that will all give the correct focal length. Any particular combination, however, may give a different amount of magnification from another combination.

When the wearer has good vision in each eye but requires different prescriptions in each eye, the resulting difference in the magnification side-effect of the different prescriptions may result in visual problems. A person who has different prescriptions has *anisometropia*. If the difference in magnification or image size caused by the different prescriptions causes visual problems, usually the breaking of fusion, then the wearer has *aniseikonia*. Specially designed lenses that attempt to correct the magnification or image size difference without changing the focal lengths of the lenses are called *iseikonic lenses* or *eikonic lenses*.

Spectacle magnification (SM) is a number that shows how much a particular lens will magnify the image on the retina. An SM of 1 means the image on the retina is the same size that it would be if the eye focused correctly with no glasses or contact lens added. An SM of 0.95 would be a 5% reduction in retinal image size; an SM of 1.05 would be a 5% increase in retinal image size.

The formula for spectacle magnification is

$$SM = \frac{1}{1 - (^t/_n) D_1} \times \frac{1}{1 - hD}$$
$$\text{(shape factor)} \qquad \text{(power factor)}$$

where t = the thickness of the lens in meters,

n = the index of refraction of the lens material,

D_1 = the base curve or front surface power of the lens,

D = the actual power of the lens,

h = the vertex distance + 3mm, converted to meters.

The first of these fractions is called the **shape factor** because it depends on the base curve selection and the thickness of the lens. Changes in base curve, lens material, and thickness affect the shape factor. The second of the fractions is called the **power factor** because it is determined by the power of the lens. Changes in vertex distance affect the power factor. The h in the power factor actually represents the distance from the back of the lens to the entrance of the pupil inside the eye, not to the apex of the cornea, which is the definition of the vertex distance. Since we cannot measure the distance to the center of the pupil, we add 3mm to the vertex distance. 3mm is used as the average distance from the corneal apex to the pupil center.

The percentage of spectacle magnification, or %SM, is found by subtracting 1 from the SM, and then multiplying by 100:

$$\%SM = (SM - 1)100$$

Therefore, an SM of 1.05 gives $\%SM = (1.05 - 1)100 = (0.05)100 = +5\%$, or 5% magnification, while a SM of +0.95 gives $\%SM = (0.95-1)100 = (-0.05)100 = -5\%$, or 5% minification.

While doing the exercises, notice that all minus lenses have a SM of less than 1, which means that they will minify the image, and all plus lenses have a SM of more than 1, which means that they will magnify the image. (Already knew that, didn't you?)

Once the determination is made that a wearer is having problems that are the result of different SM in the right and left eyes, it is necessary to estimate how much change will occur in each lens if changes are made to the shape or the vertex distance. The formulas to approximate the changes in SM are

$$\Delta\%SM = \Delta D_1 t/15$$
$$\Delta\%SM = D_1 \Delta t/15$$
$$\Delta\%SM = \Delta hD/10$$

where $\Delta\%SM$ = change in the percent of magnification,

ΔD_1 = change in front base curve only,

Δt = change in thickness only *in mm*,

t = thickness *in mm*,

Δh = change in vertex distance only *in mm*.

Note: *The symbol Δ used here symbolizes "change in." It is not a variable, nor does it refer to prism.*

Note: When using these formulas you change only one factor at a time. If you try a 1D base curve change, then use the thickness in the original problem. If you then try a 2mm thickness change, use the front curve from the original problem.

The change formulas are approximate. Changing one factor changes the others. For example, a change in base curve may change thickness and the vertex distance. On high prescriptions a change in vertex distance may require compensating the lens power (see pages 68-70.) The approximation magnification changes may be done to determine *what types of changes will be most likely to help the wearer*; then the full formula could be used with all of the proposed changes to come up with a final answer.

When changing factors that will affect magnification, do not aim to completely eliminate the differences in magnification.

EXAMPLE What is the spectacle magnification for each of the lenses in the prescription below, and what is the difference in magnification percent for the two lenses?

The Rx is: +1.50   The glasses chosen fit at 12mm. The lenses
         +4.50   are made of CR39, n = 1.498, BC's +6.25 & +9.25.

Calipering the completed lenses shows thicknesses of 3mm and 5mm.

OD

$$SM = \frac{1}{1 - (^t/_n)\,D_1} \times \frac{1}{1 - hD}$$

$$= \frac{1}{1 - (^{0.003}/_{1.498})(+6.25)} \times \frac{1}{1 - (0.015)(+1.50)}$$

$$SM = \frac{1}{1 - 0.0125167} \times \frac{1}{1 - 0.0225} = (1.01268)(1.02302) = \mathbf{1.036}$$

$$\%SM = (SM - 1)\,100 = (1.036 - 1)\,100 = \mathbf{3.6\%}$$

OS

$$SM = \frac{1}{1 - (^t/_n)\,D_1} \times \frac{1}{1 - hD}$$

$$= \frac{1}{1 - (^{0.005}/_{1.498})(+9.25)} \times \frac{1}{1 - (0.015)(+4.50)}$$

$$SM = \frac{1}{1 - 0.0308745} \times \frac{1}{1 - 0.0675} = (1.03186)(1.07239) = \mathbf{1.107}$$

$$\%SM = (SM - 1)\,100 = (1.107 - 1)\,100 = \textbf{10.7\%}$$

The right eye has 3.6% magnification, and the left eye has 10.7% magnification. The wearer has a magnification difference of $10.7 - 3.6 = \textbf{7.1\%}$.

If the wearer has good vision in each eye when corrected, then this person will probably either suppress one eye or have a problem with fusion. What can be done to decrease the 7.1% magnification difference?

1. **BC changes:** Putting both lenses on a +8.25 BC increases D_1 from +6.25 to +8.25 for the right eye, a change of +2D, and decreases D_1 from +9.25 to +8.25 for the left eye, a change of −1D.

   OD $\Delta D_1 = +2$, $\Delta SM\% = \Delta D_1 t/15 = (+2)(3) / 15 = \textbf{+0.4\% increase;}$

   With this change OD magnification would be $3.6 + 0.4 = 4.0\%$.

   OS $\Delta D_1 = -1$, $\Delta SM\% = \Delta D_1 t/15 = (-1)(5) / 15 = \textbf{−0.3\% decrease;}$

   With this change OS magnification would be $10.7 - 0.3 = 10.4\%$.
   Together, they decrease the difference from 7.1% to about **6.4%.**

Note: this may increase lens aberrations, creating other potential problems for the wearer.

2. **Thickness changes**: Make the OD 5mm thick, decrease the OS to 3mm. The right lens changes from 3mm to 5mm, a change of +2mm. The left lens changes from 5mm to 3mm, a change of −2mm.

   OD $\Delta t = +2$, $\Delta SM\% = D_1 \Delta t/15 = (+6.25)(+2) / 15 = \textbf{+0.8\% increase;}$

   With this change OD magnification would be $3.6 + 0.8 = 4.4\%$.

   OS $\Delta t = -2$, $\Delta SM\% = D_1 \Delta t/15 = (+9.25)(-2) / 15 = \textbf{−1.2\% decrease;}$

   With this change OS magnification would be $10.7 - 1.2 = 9.5\%$.
   Together, they decrease the difference from 7.1% to about 5.1%.

Note: On the OS, this change may not be safe without refitting to a smaller frame (which, if it were possible, should have been done before the whole exercise was started!).

3. **Vertex distance changes:** Move the bevel on one lens, or give the glasses co-planar misalignment, resulting in an OD VD of 13mm and OS VD of 11mm. The right lens changes from 12mm to 13mm, a change of +1mm. The left lens changes from 12mm to 11mm, a change of -1mm.

   OD $\Delta h = +1$, $\Delta SM\% = \Delta hD/10 = (+1)(+1.50) / 10 = \textbf{+0.2\% increase.}$
   With this change OD magnification would be $3.6 + 0.2 = 3.8\%$.

   OS $\Delta h = -1$, $\Delta SM\% = \Delta hD/10 = (-1)(+4.50) / 10 = \textbf{−0.5\% decrease;}$
   With this change OD magnification would be $10.7 - 0.5 = 10.2\%$.
   Together, they decrease the difference from 7.1% to about 6.4%.

Note: Bevel placement changes are more practical on minus lenses than on plus lenses.

If each of theses changes were made to the prescription, then there would seem to be a decrease from 7.1% difference to about 3.7% difference. Why?

$$OD: \quad 3.6 + 0.4 + 0.8 + 0.2 = 5.0\%;$$
$$OS \quad 10.7 - 0.3 - 1.2 - 0.5 = 8.7\%;$$
$$8.7 - 5.0 = \textbf{3.7\% difference between eyes}.$$

Reworking the original question but using the new parameters: BC's of +8.25, t = 5mm & 3mm, and VD's of 13mm and 11mm:

OD

$$SM = \cfrac{1}{1 - (^t/_n)\, D_1} \times \cfrac{1}{1 - hD}$$

$$= \cfrac{1}{1 - (^{0.005}/_{1.498})(+8.25)} \times \cfrac{1}{1 - (0.016)(+1.50)}$$

$$\mathbf{SM} = \cfrac{1}{1 - 0.0275367} \times \cfrac{1}{1 - 0.024} = (1.02832)(1.02459) = \mathbf{1.054}$$

$$\mathbf{\%SM} = (SM - 1)\,100 = (1.054 - 1)\,100 = \mathbf{5.4\%}$$

OS

$$SM = \cfrac{1}{1 - (^t/_n)\, D_1} \times \cfrac{1}{1 - hD}$$

$$= \cfrac{1}{1 - (^{0.003}/_{1.498})(+8.25)} \times \cfrac{1}{1 - (0.014)(+4.50)}$$

$$\mathbf{SM} = \cfrac{1}{1 - 0.0165220} \times \cfrac{1}{1 - 0.063} = (1.01680)(1.06724) = \mathbf{1.085}$$

$$\mathbf{\%SM} = (SM - 1)\,100 = (1.085 - 1)\,100 = \mathbf{8.5\%}$$

The right eye now has 5.4% magnification, and the left eye has 8.5% magnification, giving a difference of **3.1%** for the two eyes. Please note several items.

1. Some of these changes may not be reasonable; iseikonic lens designers rarely change all three.

2. Choosing a smaller, rounder frame that fits closer to the face may make a substantial change without the special designs. Use the original specifications, but with a VD of 8mm and thicknesses of 2.5mm and 4mm respectively, to prove this change to yourself.

3. Aspheric design lenses may also reduce the difference in SM to tolerable limits, without the special designs.

4. If the wearer could not fuse before, but decreasing the magnification difference allows binocular vision, then the cosmetics of these glasses may be perfectly acceptable to the wearer; but if the wearer suppresses one eye, or for some other reason does not notice a difference in binocular vision, the cosmetics of the iseikonic lenses may be totally unacceptable.

When computing SM for compound lenses, the magnification must be computed on each of the major meridians separately. For example, an Rx of −1.00 −4.00 x180 will have a very different magnification on the 180 meridian from what it has on the 090 meridian. The SM should be computed for the major meridian powers; in this case, for −1.00D and for −5.00D.

For all lenses, remember the following rules:

	plus lens	minus lens
increase BC	more magnification	less minification
increase t	more magnification	less minification
increase VD	more magnification	more minification

Some types of anisometropia are better corrected with contact lenses, others with glasses. Not everyone with anisometropia gets aniseikonia from their glasses, so iseikonic lenses would only be considered if the wearer is having problems connected to magnification changes. There are several tools other than the formulas to use to help design iseikonic lenses, and numerous factors to consider before becoming involved in designing iseikonic lenses. A very complete discussion of this problem and the potential solutions may be found in Fannin and Grosvenor, *Clinical Optics, 2nd Ed.*, pages 300-325.

SPECTACLE MAGNIFICATION EXERCISES
(Round all magnification percents to one decimal place.)

1. The Rx is OD −14.50 OS −10.00. Center thickness is 1.5mm OU, material is polycarbonate (n = 1.586), fitting vertex distance 9mm, BC +1.50 OU. What is the SM for each eye, and the difference between the eyes? What could be done to decrease the difference? Try:
    a. Increasing the center thickness of the OD by 1mm.
    b. Moving the bevel placement on the OS to increase the VD by 2mm and on the OD to decrease the VD by 1mm.
    c. Increasing the BC one diopter for OD, decreasing one diopter for OS.
    Which changes make the most difference? Are they practical? (Not coming up with the answers at the end of the section? Remember to add 3mm to the VD but not to the change in VD, and watch the signs in the denominators.)

2. What is the SM for contact lenses (VD = 0) for the prescription OD +1.50, OS +4.50? For contact lenses, the shape factor is essentially 1, so we use only the power factor. The vertex distance is 0mm. Notice that this is the same prescription used for the example on page 131. Compare the difference in magnification from glasses to contact lenses.

THOMPSON'S FORMULA FOR OBLIQUELY CROSSED CYLINDERS

What happens if an aphake has an Rx that says "overrefracted OD +1.25 −1.25 x113" for glasses that have an Rx of +12.50 −2.25 x085? Or, overrefraction of a new contact lens wearer gives −1.25 −2.00 x015 on a lens that is −5.00 −1.00 x180? If the two Rx's being combined are at the same axis or are 90 degrees apart, transpose if necessary to put both Rx's in the same axis, add the sphere powers for the new sphere, and add the cylinder powers for the new cylinder. If the axis are not 90 degrees apart, the practical way to solve this problem is to dot a lens with the overrefraction Rx on axis, place it and the glasses in the focimeter at the same time, and neutralize the result. But this book is a formulas reference, so we will use formulas!

First, transpose the Rx's to plus cylinder. (Transposing is not strictly necessary, but will make the calculations "easier".) Label the Rx with the *lower value axis* S_1 C_1 x a_1, and the other S_2 C_2 x a_2. The angle γ is $a_2 - a_1$.

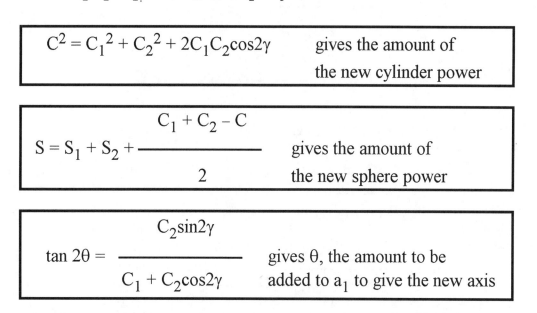

$$C^2 = C_1^2 + C_2^2 + 2C_1C_2\cos2\gamma \qquad \text{gives the amount of the new cylinder power}$$

$$S = S_1 + S_2 + \frac{C_1 + C_2 - C}{2} \qquad \text{gives the amount of the new sphere power}$$

$$\tan 2\theta = \frac{C_2\sin2\gamma}{C_1 + C_2\cos2\gamma} \qquad \text{gives } \theta, \text{ the amount to be added to } a_1 \text{ to give the new axis}$$

If the result is a negative axis, remember that what is on the lower half of the lens is the same as what is 180 degrees away on the upper half. Just add 180 to the negative answer to find the new prescription axis. Or, if the resulting axis is over 180, subtract 180 from it.

EXAMPLE 1:   The current Rx in the glasses is   OS +10.50 +2.00 x015
   The overrefraction is   −0.50 +0.75 x045.
   What lens power should be ordered?
Step 1. Put the prescriptions in plus cylinder form. Label the Rx with the lower value axis as S_1 C_1 x a_1 and the other as S_2 C_2 x a_2.

The Rx's are in + cylinder form, and are in the correct order. So:

$$S_1 = +10.50 \qquad\qquad S_2 = -0.50$$
$$C_1 = +2.00 \qquad\qquad C_2 = +0.75$$
$$a_1 = 015 \qquad\qquad a_2 = 045$$

Step 2. The angle γ is $a_2 - a_1 = 45 - 15 = 30$; $2\gamma = 60$

Step 3. Compute the new cylinder power.

$$C^2 = C_1{}^2 + C_2{}^2 + 2C_1C_2\cos2\gamma$$
$$= (2.00)^2 + (0.75)^2 + 2(2.00)(0.75)(\cos60)$$
$$= 4 + 0.5625 + (3)(0.5) = 6.0625$$

$$\mathbf{C = \sqrt{6.0625} = +2.46, \text{ the new cylinder power}}$$

Step 4. Compute the new sphere power.

$$S = S_1 + S_2 + \frac{C_1 + C_2 - C}{2}$$

$$= +10.50 - 0.50 + \frac{2 + 0.75 - 2.46}{2} = +10.00 + 0.145$$

$$\mathbf{S = +10.15, \text{ the new sphere power}}$$

Step 5. Compute the new axis.

$$\tan2\theta = \frac{C_2\sin2\gamma}{C_1 + C_2\cos2\gamma}$$

$$\tan2\theta = \frac{(0.75)\sin60}{(2) + (0.75)\cos60} = \frac{0.6495}{2.375} = 0.27347$$

so $2\theta = 15.29$, and $\theta = 7.6$ which rounds to 8 degrees. The 8 degree change is added to a_1; so $15 + 8 = \mathbf{23, \text{ the new axis}}$.

The combined Rx is now +10.15 +2.46 x023. This answer, changed to the nearest eighth so that it may be ordered or surfaced, is **+10.12 +2.50 x023.**

This set of formulas comes in a variety of forms in different textbooks. The problems may also be solved graphically, using vector analysis. Possible sources are Fannin and Grosvenor, *Clinical Optics, 2nd Ed.*, pages 43-48; Epting and Morgret, *Ophthalmic Mechanics and Dispensing*, pages 106-110; and Jalie, *The Principles of Ophthalmic Lenses, 4th Ed.*, pages 287-296. What is shown here seems to be the easiest combination of several different versions.

EXAMPLE 2: Rx is +12.50 -3.50 x180. Over refraction is +1.75 -1.00 x135. What should be ordered?

Step 1. transpose and rearrange: +0.75 + 1.00 x045

                                        +9.00 + 3.50 x090

$$S_1 = +0.75 \qquad S_2 = +9.00$$
$$C_1 = +1.00 \qquad C_2 = +3.50$$
$$a_1 = 045 \qquad a_2 = 090$$

Step 2. $\gamma = 45, \quad 2\gamma = 90$

Step 3. $C^2 = C_1^2 + C_2^2 + 2C_1C_2\cos2\gamma$

$$= (1.00)^2 + (3.50)^2 + 2(1.00)(3.50)(\cos90)$$
$$= 1 + 12.25 + (2)(3.5)(0) = 13.25$$

$$C = \sqrt{13.25} = +3.64, \textbf{ the new cylinder power}$$

Step 4.

$$S = S_1 + S_2 + \frac{C_1 + C_2 - C}{2}$$

$$= +0.75 + 9.00 + \frac{1 + 3.50 - 3.64}{2} = +9.75 + 0.43$$

$$S = +10.18, \textbf{ the new sphere power}$$

Step 5.

$$\tan 2\theta = \frac{C_2\sin2\gamma}{C_1 + C_2\cos2\gamma}$$

$$\tan 2\theta = \frac{(3.5)\sin90}{(1) + (3.5)\cos90} = \frac{3.5}{1} = 3.5$$

so $2\theta = 74$, and $\theta = 37$ degrees. The 37 degree change is added to a_1;

so 45 + 37 = **82, the new axis**.

The new Rx is +10.18 +3.64 x082, or +13.82 -3.64 x172. Changed to eighths so that it may be ordered or surfaced, it is **+13.87 -3.62 x172.**

OBLIQUELY CROSSED CYLINDERS EXERCISE

Combine −6.50 −2.00 x054 with −1.50 −0.75 x010. (Remember: Start by transposing to plus cylinder form.)

FRESNEL'S EQUATION FOR REFLECTION

    When a light ray travels from one transparent material to another material, one of three things happen: it is refracted, which was discussed in Section II, or it is absorbed, which will be discussed on pages 142-147, or it is reflected. The Frenchman Fresnel, also known for lighthouse beacons and what has become press-on optics, determined that the amount of incident light reflected from the interface between two transparent materials depends solely on the refractive indices of the two materials.

The percentage of incident light that is reflected from a transparent surface is equal to

$$100 \; \frac{(n_r - n_i)^2}{(n_r + n_i)^2}$$

where n_i is the index of refraction of the material that the light is traveling from, n_r is the index of refraction of the material that the light is entering.

Since the difference in the numerator is squared, the percent of incident light reflected from the surface is the same for light entering or leaving the lens, so the order in which n_i and n_r are listed is not important.

The version of this equation that we use when the lens is in air is

$$100 \; \frac{(n - 1)^2}{(n + 1)^2}$$

where n is the index of refraction of the lens material.

If I_0 is the intensity of light falling on a lens, then the amount of light entering the lens will be I_1, which is I_0 – the amount reflected. Thus:

$$I_1 = I_0 - I_0 \times \frac{(n - 1)^2}{(n + 1)^2}$$

I_1 is the intensity of light that travels through the non-absorptive lens to the back surface of the lens. I_2, then, will be what is not reflected from the back surface of the lens, and therefore exits the lens through the back surface.

$$I_2 = I_1 - I_1 \times \frac{(n - 1)^2}{(n + 1)^2}$$

EXAMPLE: What percentage of the incident light is transmitted through a white (or clear) lens made of crown glass?

I_0 will be 100% of the incident light.
n = 1.523.

$$\frac{(n - 1)^2}{(n + 1)^2} = \frac{(0.523)^2}{(2.523)^2} = \frac{0.2735}{6.3655} = 0.043$$

100 (0.043) = 4.3% of the incident light reflects from the front surface of the lens.

Or, given that 0.043 of the light reflects from the surface,

$I_0 = 100\%$

$I_1 = I_0 - I_0(\text{reflection}) = I_0 - I_0(0.043) = 100 - (100)(0.043) = 95.7\%$

$I_2 = I_1 - I_1(\text{reflection}) = I_1 - I_1(0.043) = 95.7 - 95.7(0.043)$

$= 95.7 - 4.1 = \mathbf{91.6\%.}$

In words, what the formula tells us is that 100% − 4.3% = 95.7% of the incident light travels into the lens. Since the lens is white, or clear, all of this light reaches the back surface of the lens. 4.3% of the light reaching the back of the lens is reflected back into the lens. So (0.043) (95.7%) = 4.1% of the light reflects from the back surface. 95.7% − 4.1% = 91.6% of the incident light actually travels through the lens.

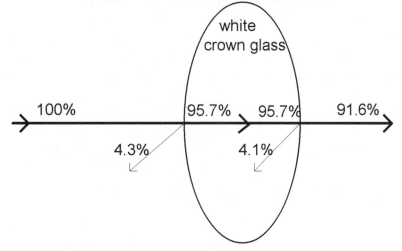

Now take the same lens and immerse it in water. Of the light traveling through the water, the amount that reflects from the first surface is

$$\frac{(n_1 - n_2)^2}{(n_1 + n_2)^2} = \frac{(1.523 - 1.33)^2}{(1.523 + 1.33)^2} = \frac{(0.193)^2}{(2.853)^2} = 0.0046, \text{ or } 0.5\%$$

One-half of one percent of the incident light reflects from the front surface, so 99.5% of the light enters the lens. (0.005) (99.5%) = 0.5% more of the original light traveling through the water reflects back into the lens, leaving 99% of the incident light to travel through the lens back into the water. Why do you suppose it is harder to see a clear lens in water than in air? If you do not believe it, drop a clear uncoated lens into a fish tank.

REFLECTION EXERCISES

1. What percent of incident light is reflected from the front surface of a clear CR39 lens? What percentage of the original incident light reflects back into the lens from the back surface? What percentage of the incident light is transmitted through the lens?

2. What percent of incident light is reflected from the front and back surfaces of a polycarbonate lens? What percentage of the incident light is transmitted completely through the polycarbonate lens?

3. Do the calculations again for a high index lens material with index of refraction of 1.66. Do you see the trend? Why do reflections bother high-index wearers more than CR39 wearers, regardless of prescription?

ANTI-REFLECTIVE COATINGS

Two conditions should be met for an anti-reflective coating to work at its best. The first condition is that the amount of light reflected from the coating should be equal to the amount of light reflected from the lens. The second condition is that the wave of light reflected from the coating should cancel the wave of light reflected from the lens. (These conditions assume that the amplitudes of the incident and reflected waves are equal.)

If the *index of refraction of the coating material is equal to the square root of the index of refraction of the lens material,* then the exact same amount of light will reflect from the surface of the coating and from the interface between the coating and the lens material. Since the coating must have several other attributes, such as being insoluble in water, the best coating materials do not meet this criterion exactly.

> When the coating index = square root of lens material index
> then the reflections from the coating surface and the lens surface
> have equal intensity.

Two waves traveling exactly out of phase with each other cancel each other, or have *destructive interference.*

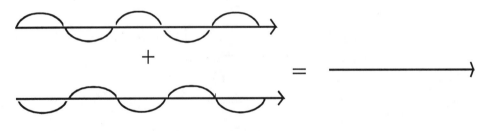

Two waves traveling in phase with each other compound each other. They have *constructive interference.*

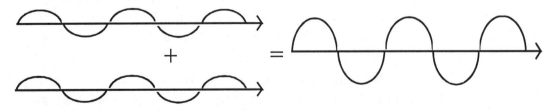

If the thickness of the lens coating is 1/4 of the wavelength of the incident light, then the reflections from the coating and from the lens will cancel each other, or have destructive interference.

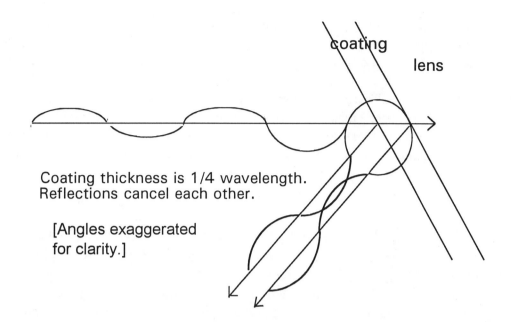

Coating thickness is 1/4 wavelength.
Reflections cancel each other.

[Angles exaggerated
for clarity.]

If the thickness of the lens coating is 1/2 of the wavelength of the incident light, then the reflections from the coating and the lens will compound each other. They have constructive interference.

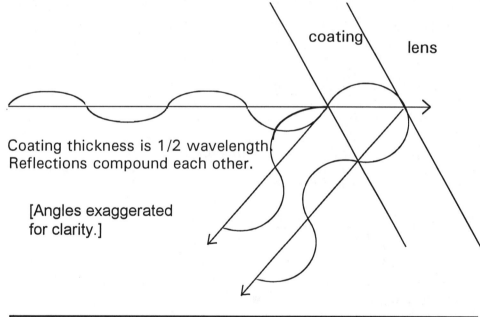

Coating thickness is 1/2 wavelength.
Reflections compound each other.

[Angles exaggerated
for clarity.]

When the thickness of coating = $1/4\lambda$ or $3/4\lambda$ or $5/4\lambda$ or ....
reflections cancel, or have *destructive interference*.

The diagrams and rule of thumb are extremely simplistic representations of what happens. The optics sections in some college physics textbooks or advanced optical theory books go into more detail about the mechanics of the reflections. What is important to us is that the coating thickness should be an odd multiple of 1/4 of the wavelength of the incoming light. Most manufacturers use $1/4\lambda$.

The visible spectrum ranges from about 380nm to about 760nm. One-fourth of 760nm is 190nm. But 190nm is 1/2 of 380nm. So the coating thickness that would cancel the high end red waves would also compound the low end violet waves. Likewise, for any wavelength between, the coating that would cancel one color will at least partially compound other colors. Therefore, coating manufacturers apply several layers of varying thickness in order to cancel a majority of the reflected light waves. The colored sheen that is seen on anti-reflective coatings is what is left based on a particular manufacturer' combination of coatings and thicknesses. Each AR manufacturer is careful to keep the resulting colored sheen consistent from batch to batch.

TRANSMISSION THROUGH ABSORPTIVE LENSES

Once a light ray enters the front surface of lens, it can be either absorbed by the lens material or transmitted through to the back surface of the lens.

Making absorptive lenses from CR39 and other plastic materials requires dyeing the lenses. By immersing the lens in a warm dye bath, pigments that will absorb some of the incident light are incorporated into the lens material in an even layer less than 1/2mm thick. Thus, the absorption of light does not depend on the thickness of the lens, only on the amount of pigment absorbed by the material. A lens that has been dyed to a 15% absorption transmits 85% of the entering light. For an uncoated CR39 lens, 4.0% of the incident light is reflected from the front surface, so $I_1 = 96\%$.

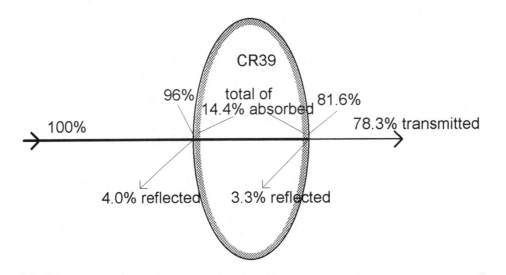

If 85% of the light entering the lens is transmitted, then $(0.85)(96) = 81.6\%$ of the incident light is transmitted to the back surface of the lens. Since the lens is uncoated, 4% of 81.6% will be reflected back into the lens at the back surface. $(0.04)(81.6) = 3.3\%$ is reflected at the back surface. $81.6 - 3.3 = 78.3\%$ of the original light falling on the lens is actually transmitted through the lens. (See the discussion of Fresnel's equation for reflection, pages 137-140.)

Sometimes white (or clear) glass lenses are given an absorptive coating. When this process is performed the transmission as shown above works the same way. A lens' absorptive ability is indicated as one number, regardless of whether the absorption occurs at one surface or both surfaces. In the lens above, the 15% absorption occurs partially at the front and partially at the back surface. A 15% absorptive coating on a glass lens would be all absorbed at the surface that is coated. In either case 100% − 15% = 85% of the light entering the lens is transmitted through the lens.

Most absorptive *glass* lenses are not coated. Instead they have the absorptive oxides distributed evenly throughout the glass material. The absorptive rating for the glass material is indicated by a percent per 2mm thickness. Every 2mm of lens material that the incident light travels through absorbs more light. The transmission rating for the material is 100 − absorption rating per 2mm of thickness.

In the following exercises sometimes the amounts of light will be expressed as decimals, and sometimes as percents. Convert from one to the other by multiplying or dividing by 100. Therefore, $0.56 \Rightarrow 56\%$; $82\% \Rightarrow 0.82$. Round the numbers to one decimal in percent or three decimals in decimal form. When *adding* or *subtracting*, have BOTH numbers in either decimal or percent form. When *multiplying*, either use both numbers in decimal form (the answer will be in decimal form) or have one in percent and one in decimal (the answer will be in percent form).

EXAMPLE 1: What is the total transmission through the center of a crown glass lens with 15% absorption per 2mm of thickness, if the center thickness of the lens is 6mm?

1. The reflection from the front surface is **4.3%**, or 100% − 4.3% = **95.7%** of the incident light enters the lens. (See the discussion of Fresnel's equation for reflection, pages 137-140.)

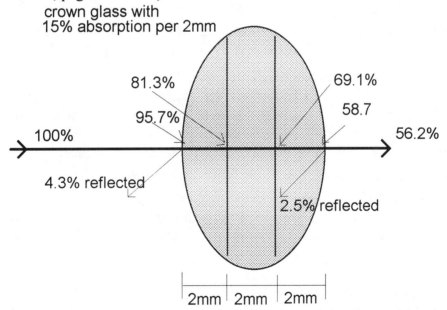

crown glass with
15% absorption per 2mm

2. The first 2mm of the lens absorbs 15% of the light that reaches it, or it transmits 85% ⇒ 0.85 of the light reaching it. (0.85)(95.7) = **81.3%** of the incident light is transmitted through the first 2mm of thickness of the lens.

3. 15% of the 81.3% will be absorbed in the next 2mm of lens, or 85% ⇒ 0.85 of the 81.3% will be transmitted. (0.85)(81.3) = **69.1%** of the incident light is transmitted through the second 2mm of thickness of the lens.

4. 15% of the 69.1% will be absorbed in the last 2mm of the lens, or 85% $\Rightarrow$ 0.85 of the 69.1% will be transmitted. $(0.85)(69.1) =$ **58.7%** of the incident light is transmitted through to the back surface of the lens.

5. 4.3% of the light reaching the back of the lens is reflected back into the lens, or 95.7% $\Rightarrow$ 0.957 will pass through the back surface. $(0.957)(58.7) =$ **56.2% of the incident light is transmitted through the lens at the center**.

Notice that the 15% absorptive CR39 lens allowed 78% of the incident light through the lens, which is about what will be transmitted through this glass lens at the 2mm edge; but the center of the 15% absorptive glass lens allowed just over 1/2 of the incident light through. (Just what you would have expected, isn't it?)

Lambert's equation for lens transmission will determine the absorption of the glass lens in fewer steps. Let q = thickness/2 (in mm). In the lens above, q = 6 / 2 = 3. Let T be the amount of incident light transmitted per 2mm thickness. Then the amount of light transmitted through the lens from front surface to back surface is

$$\boxed{I_2 = I_1 T^q}$$

where I_2 = intensity of light reaching the back surface of the lens,

I_1 = intensity of light entering the lens,

T = the transmission factor per 2mm of lens thickness, (in decimal form)

q = the thickness of the lens in mm divided by 2mm.

In example 1, I_1 = 95.7%, T = 100% − 15% = 85% = 0.85, and q = 6mm/2mm = 3. So the amount of light transmitted to the back surface of the lens is

$$I_2 = (95.7)(0.85)^3 = (95.7)(0.614) = 58.8\%$$

which is what the computations above gave. (The 0.01% difference is the result of rounding when we did the transmission step-by-step.) Use the transmission in decimal form for this equation. (The reflection from the back surface still needs to be computed.)

What if the thickness of the lens is 4.7mm? Now q = 4.7 / 2 = 2.35. How will you do this with your calculator? If your calculator has the sin/cos/tan functions, then somewhere on it there is a key labeled either x^y or y^x. (If your calculator *also* has a key labeled x^n or y^n, do *not* use this key.) Enter the transmission amount, in the above example 0.85, press the x^y or y^x key, enter 2.35, press =. The result is 0.68255.... What you are doing when you enter this sequence is telling the calculator what x is, then that you want to raise it to the y power, then what y is.

Ready for another example?

EXAMPLE 2: An uncoated crown glass lens has an absorptive rating of 25%/2mm of thickness. The lens is ground to an Rx of −5.00D, with a center thickness of 2.2mm. What is the transmission through the center of the lens? If the lens edge calipers to 7.1mm, what is the transmission through the thickest edge of the lens?

1. The reflection from the front surface at both the center and the edge will be 4.3%, so **95.7%** of the incident light will enter the lens.

2. At the center of the lens, thickness = 2.2mm, q = 2.2/2 = 1.1, and T = 100 − 25 = 75% = 0.75. The transmission through the lens at the center is
$$I_2 = (95.7)(0.75)^{1.1} = (95.7)(0.729) = \textbf{69.7\%}$$

3. 4.3% = 0.043 of the 69.7% of the incident light that reached the back surface at the center of the lens is reflected back into the lens at the back surface. So (69.7)(0.43) = 3.0% of the incident light is reflected, leaving 69.7 − 3.0 = **66.7% transmission through the center of the lens.**

4. At the edge of the lens, thickness = 7.1, q = 7.1 / 2 = 3.55, and T = 100 − 25 = 75% = 0.75, and 95.7% of the incident light enters the lens at the edge. So the transmission to the back surface of the lens is
$$I_2 = (95.7)(0.75)^{3.55} = (95.7)(0.3601) = \textbf{34.5\%}$$

5. 4.3% = 0.043 of the 34.5% of the incident light that reached the back surface at the edge of the lens is reflected back into the lens at the back surface. So (34.5)(0.043) = 1.5% of the incident light is reflected, leaving 34.5 − 1.5 = **33.0% transmission through the edge of the lens.**

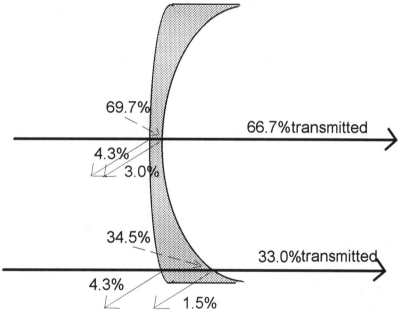

You already knew that the edge would be a lot darker than the center, didn't you?

Photochromatic lenses do not lend themselves to the use of Lambert's equation. Plastic photochromatics have a thin layer of photoreactive material on the front surface of the lens, and so they have an even distribution of absorption over the surface of the lens, regardless of lens thickness. Photochromatic glass has silver halide mixed evenly throughout the material, so it seems that it would work the way absorptive glass works. However, the amount of transmission or absorption depends on the amount of UV light reaching the silver halide. Since the UV rays are absorbed by the change in the lens material, the transmission of UV decreases as the ray penetrates the lens. Therefore the amount of change in the lens material decreases as the ray penetrates the lens. In the full dark state, the innermost 2mm of a thick lens does not absorb as much light as the outer 2mm absorbed.

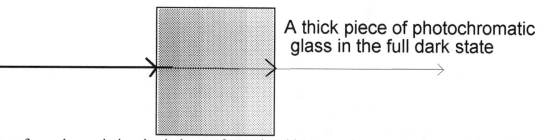

A thick piece of photochromatic glass in the full dark state

Therefore, the variation in darkness from the thinnest point on the lens to the thickest point on the lens is not as great as the variation in darkness on a non-variable absorptive glass lens.

Finally, look at what happens when several absorptive lenses are lined up in a row. If the total transmission through the first lens is 75%, and the total transmission through the second lens is 50%, the total transmission through the two lenses will be 50% = 0.50 of 75%, or (0.5)(75) = 37.5%. Consider a person driving in a car with tinted windshields. If the windshield has a total transmission of 80%, and the driver is wearing sunglasses with a total transmission of 20%, the driver is actually seeing (0.20)(80) = 16% of the incident light. What if the same driver wears lenses with a 30% – 0% gradient tint when driving at night? If the person drives looking through the top of the lenses (most of us do) where the transmission is 70%, then the driver is receiving (0.80)(70) = 56% of the incident light. 56% transmission is too much to "help" with car headlights, but may very well result in not seeing objects or beings in the low-light low-contrast conditions at the side of the road.

TRANSMISSION EXERCISES
(Round answers to one-tenth of a percent.)

1. What is the total transmission through a plastic lens having an index of refraction of 1.66, tinted with a 15% cosmetic tint?

2. What is the total transmission through an anti-reflective coated glass lens having an absorptive rating of 15% per 2mm thickness? The glass lens has a center thickness of 2.2mm and the thickest edge is 5.7mm. (Since the lens is AR coated, you may ignore surface reflections.)

3. Suppose a plano photochromatic lens has an absorptive rating of 18% in its unexposed state, and 56% in the car during the day. If the lens is not AR-coated, and the wearer is driving a car with windshields tinted to 15% absorption, what is the total transmission to the driver in bright sunlight? What is the total transmission at night? (Assume that the index of refraction for the photochromatic glass and for the windshield are both 1.523.) Steps:
    a. Determine the final transmission through the car windshield, index 1.523, absorption 15%. (Keep in decimal form.)
    b. Determine the final transmission through the photochromatic lens only, with 56% absorption, and index 1.523. (Keep in decimal form.)
    c. Multiply the two final transmission numbers from part a and b. Convert to a percent. This is how much of the incident light this wearer sees while driving during the day.

Optical Formulas Tutorial

d. Determine the final transmission through the photochromatic lens only, with 18% absorption, and index 1.523. (Keep in decimal form.)

e. Multiply the two final transmission numbers from part a and d. Convert to a percent. This is how much of the incident light this wearer sees while driving at night.

POLARIZING FILTERS

Normal diffuse sunlight contains waves that are vibrating in every direction perpendicular to the direction of travel of the sunlight. The light beam is said to be **unpolarized** if it contains waves oscillating in random directions. The light beam is said to be **polarized** if it contains waves oscillating on or near only one plane.

LIGHT BEAMS TRAVELING PERPENDICULAR TO THE PAGE

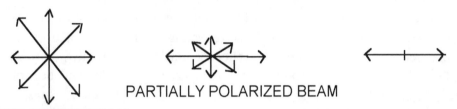

PARTIALLY POLARIZED BEAM

UNPOLARIZED BEAM
rays vibrating in all directions

LINEARLY POLARIZED BEAM
rays vibrating in only one direction

There are essentially two main ways of limiting the light in a light beam to oscillate on only one plane. A beam of unpolarized light can be **polarized** by reflection from the surface of a material that does not conduct electricity (a dielectric material.) Examples of dielectric, or non-conducting, materials are water, snow, sand, glass, and pavement. Or the beam can be polarized by passing it through a material with a crystalline structure that only allows transmission of rays vibrating in a particular direction. Examples of crystals that polarize transmitted light are quartz, tourmaline, and iodine in a particular compound or matrix. Iodine impregnated in a sheet of polyvinyl alcohol is used in ophthalmic polarizing lenses.

A beam of light that is completely polarized, so that all rays are oscillating in only one direction, is called **linearly polarized**, or **plane polarized.** (Physicists prefer linearly polarized because there is also a circular polarization, which will not be discussed here.) A beam of light that is not completely polarized is called **partially polarized.** The light that reflects from the surface of water is partially polarized, unless the angle of incidence of the rays of light satisfy **Brewster's Equation**:

$$\boxed{\tan i = n_i/n_r}$$

where i is the angle of incidence of the incident light,

  n_i is the index of the incident material,

  n_r is the index of the reflecting material.

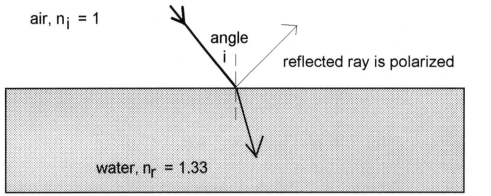

air, n_i = 1

angle i

reflected ray is polarized

water, n_r = 1.33

For a pond sitting out in the sunshine of mid-morning or mid-afternoon, n_i = 1, n_r = 1.33. Brewster's formula gives

tan i = n/n_r = 1/1.33=0.7519; therefore i = 37°.

When the sun is at an angle of 37° with the normal to the surface of the water (which means 53° up from the horizon), the light reflecting from the surface of the water is linearly polarized. At any other angle the reflected sunshine is partially polarized.

Unpolarized light passing through a polarizing crystal or film will be polarized. If polarized light passes through a second polarizing film, the final total transmission depends on the relationship between the axes of the two filters. If the second filter is oriented in the same direction as the axis of the first filter, all of the light that passes through the first will pass through the second. (We are ignoring the surface reflections and the absorbing pigments present in the filter material.) If the axis of the second filter is at 90° to the first, none of the polarized light will emerge from the second filter. At any other orientation, the percent of the polarized light that is transmitted through the second filter can be found from *Malus' law*:

$$I_2 = I_1 \cos^2 \theta$$

where I_1 is the intensity of light emerging from the first filter,

I_2 is the intensity of light emerging from the second filter,

θ is the angle between the axis of the two filters.

$\cos^2 0°$ = 1, so when the filters have their axis oriented in the same direction, $I_2 = I_1$. $\cos^2 90°$ = 0, so when the filters are at 90 degrees to each other I_2 = 0. In these two situations the equation verifies what you already knew. If the filters are at 30° to each other, $I_2 = I_1 \cos^2 30 = I_1 \times 0.75$, or 75% of the light traveling through the first filter will travel through the second filter. If the filters are at 45° to each other, 50% of the light transmitted through the first filter will be transmitted through the second filter.

When unpolarized light passes through one linearly polarizing filter, 50% of the incident light is transmitted through the single filter regardless of the orientation of the filter. If 50% of the incident light passes through the first filter, and the second filter is held with the polarizer at 45° to the first, then (0.50)(50%)=25% of the originally incident light passes through the two filters.

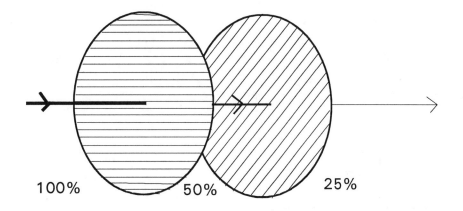

100%   50%   25%

What happens when three polarizing filters are in a row, with the axis of the second 45° from the axis of the *first* filter, and the axis of the third 90° from the axis of the *first* filter? It seems that no light should go through, since the first and third are at 90°. But, according to Malus' law, 50% of what travels through the first filter will travel through the second filter, and 50% of what travels through the second filter will travel through the third filter. As a result, placing a second filter between the first and third filters means that 12.5% of the light that was incident on the first filter will be transmitted through the third filter.

POLARIZATION EXERCISES

1. What is Brewster's angle (in air) for crown glass, n = 1.523?

2. What percentage of incident light will emerge from a series of four polarizing filters, each at 30° to the one before?

3. What common piece of ophthalmic laboratory equipment uses Malus' law?

DIFFRACTION

Diffraction is the bending of waves when they pass the edge of a very small slit. This is easy to infer as a result of wave motion; it is not easy to explain using rays without a wave nature to describe light. Its apparent absence was the major reason that the wave theory of light was ignored for centuries.

barrier with an opening

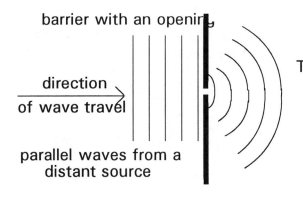

direction
of wave travel

parallel waves from a
distant source

The edges of the wave emerg
from behind the barrier diver
as if the edges of the waves
originated at the barrier

It was not until the early 1800s that Thomas Young used very small slits and near-monochromatic light to demonstrate that the waves do bend, and that interference and augmentation of light waves occurs when several small slits are next to each other. Using the method shown below plus some trigonometry, it is possible to compute the actual wavelength of the monochromatic light wave.

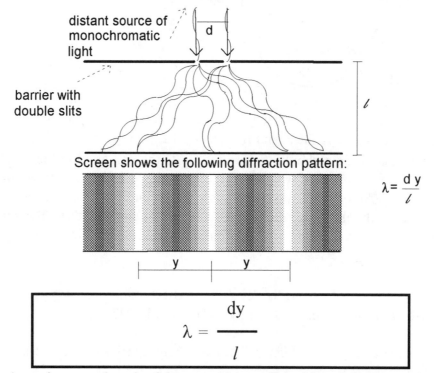

$$\lambda = \frac{dy}{l}$$

where λ = wavelength of the monochromatic incident light,
        d = distance between the slits on the diffraction grating, in meters,
        y = distance between the first two areas of constructive interference,
        l = distance from the diffraction grating to the screen.

EXAMPLE: A beam of monochromatic light from a speaker's laser pointer passes through a diffraction grating with slits that are spaced at 500 per mm. The diffraction grating is 10cm away from the screen. If the distance between the first two areas of constructive interference is 35mm, what is the wavelength of the light? What color is the laser beam?

The formula is $\lambda = \frac{dy}{l}$.

Step 1: Since the slits are spaces at 500 per millimeter, there are 500,000 slits per meter. Therefore, the spacing between the slits, d, is 1/500,000 = 0.000002 = 2×10^{-6}m.

Step 2: y = 35mm = 0.035m = 3.5×10^{-2}m

Step 3: l = 10cm = 0.1m

Therefore: $\lambda = \frac{dy}{l} = (2\times10^{-6})(3.5\times10^{-2})/(0.1) = 7\times10^{-8}/0.1 = 70\times10^{-8}$

$= 700\times10^{-9}$m = 700nm, which is a deep red light wave.

DIFFRACTION EXERCISE

1. What is the wavelength of a monochromatic beam of light if, when it is passed through a grating having slits that are 600 per mm, the distance between the first two areas of constructive interference is 33cm when the screen on which the interference pattern is projected is 10cm away? What color is the beam of light?

BACK AND FRONT VERTEX POWER

The nominal power of a lens is the sum of the two surface powers. When a lens is thick, the nominal power is not accurate. If the surface powers are substantially different from each other, the order of the surfaces as well as the thickness of the lens will have an effect on the power of the lens.

The **back vertex power** is the power measured at the back of the ophthalmic lens, is what the wearer sees, and is what is normally measured in the focimeter (or lensometer). In a meniscus lens having one convex side and one concave side, we consider the front of the lens to be the convex side of the lens.

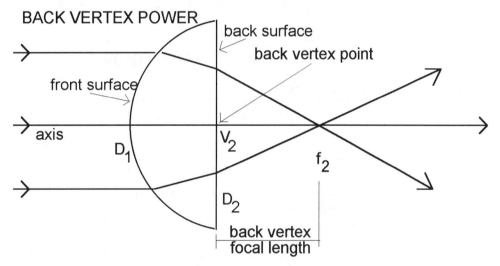

The formula for the *back vertex power* of the lens is

$$D_B = \frac{D_1}{1 - (^t/_n)\, D_1} + D_2$$

where D_1=front surface power,

D_2=back surface power,

t = thickness between the front and back vertices of the lens, in meters,

n = index of refraction for the lens material.

Note: The back vertex of the lens is the point where the axis of the lens intersects the back surface of the lens. The focal length based on this definition of back vertex power is the distance from the back vertex of the lens to the secondary focal point.

The *front vertex power*, also called the **neutralizing power**, is the power found when the ray is incident first on the back side of the lens. The front vertex power is often used by contact lens manufacturers, who will list it as the *FVP*. To measure the front vertex power in the focimeter, place the lens with the front surface toward the lens stop instead of the back surface. We use the difference between the distance and near front vertex powers to determine the add power of any bifocal segment that is molded or fused to the front surface of the lens.

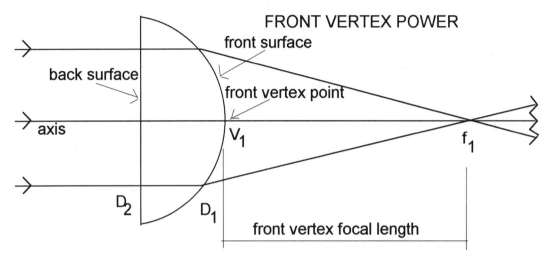

The formula for the *front vertex power* of the lens is

$$D_F = \frac{D_2}{1 - (^t/_n) D_2} + D_1$$

where D_1 = front surface power,

D_2 = back surface power,

t = thickness between the front and back vertices of the lens, in meters,

n = index of refraction for the lens material.

Note: The front vertex of the lens is the point where the axis of the lens intersects the front surface of the lens. The focal length based on this definition of front vertex power is the distance from the front vertex of the lens to the first focal point.

Looking at the diagrams, for the back vertex power the ray enters D_1 first, then travels the thickness of the lens, then exits D_2. Therefore, it is the surface power of the front of the lens that is affected by the thickness of the lens, so the back vertex power formula adjusts the power of D_1. Likewise, the front vertex power formula adjusts the power of D_2 because the thickness of the lens affects the bending that occurs at the back of the lens.

The *equivalent power* of the lens is determined using the formula

$$D = D_1 + D_2 - [^t/_n]D_1 D_2.$$

The equivalent power is actually the way to locate the principal planes for a thick lens, and will be discussed on page 170. A variation on the equivalent power formula is sometimes used for an *approximation* of the back and front vertex powers:

$$\boxed{\begin{aligned} D_B &\approx D_1 + D_2 + (^t/_n)(D_1)^2 \\ D_F &\approx D_1 + D_2 + (^t/_n)(D_2)^2 \end{aligned}}$$

EXAMPLE: Find the front and back vertex powers of a thick lens with surface curves of +12.00 and −3.00, a center thickness of 14mm, made of CR39, n=1.498.

$$D_B = \frac{D_1}{1 - (^t/_n)\,D_1} + D_2$$

$$= \frac{+12.00}{1 - (^{0.014}/_{1.498})\,(+12.00)} + (-3.00)$$

$$= (+12.00) / (0.8879) - 3.00 = +13.52 - 3.00$$

$$\mathbf{D_B = +10.52D}$$

$$D_F = \frac{D_2}{1 - (^t/_n)\,D_2} + D_1$$

$$= \frac{-3.00}{1 - (^{0.014}/_{1.498})\,(-3.00)} + (+12.00)$$

$$= (-3.00) / (1.0280) + 12.00 = -2.92 + 12.00$$

$$\mathbf{D_F = +9.08D}$$

Approximation formula:

$$D_B \approx D_1 + D_2 + (^t/_n)(D_1)^2$$
$$= +12.00 + (-3.00) + (^{0.014}/_{1.498})(+12.00)^2$$

$$\mathbf{D_B} \approx +9.00 + 1.35 = \mathbf{+10.35D}$$

$$D_F \approx D_1 + D_2 + (^t/_n)(D_2)^2$$
$$= +12.00 + (-3.00) + (^{0.014}/_{1.498})(-3.00)^2$$

$$\mathbf{D_F} \approx +9.00 + 0.08 = \mathbf{+9.08D}$$

Note: +10.52 is what the lens will read in the focimeter (or lensometer) and is what the wearer will experience (ignoring vertex distance). The powers are not changed to 1/8 diopter steps because they are actual effective powers: they will not be ordered from a lab or noted in the wearer's records.

VERTEX POWER EXERCISES
(Round to hundredths of a diopter.)

What are the back and front vertex powers of the following lenses?

1. $D_1 = +6.50$

    $D_2 = -6.50$

    $t = 2mm$

    $n = 1.50$

2. $D_1 = +10.25$

    $D_2 = -5.25$

    $t = 6mm$

    $n = 1.60$

3. $D_1 = +12.50$

    $D_2 = -2.50$

    $t = 9mm$

    $n = 1.586$

SECTION VII: IMAGE FORMATION

IMAGE SIZE AND PLACEMENT: MIRRORS

In Section II we discussed the law of reflection, which states that the angle of incidence is equal to the angle of reflection. Reflection from a plane mirror will change the direction of a ray of light, but will not change the *vergence* of two rays, meaning the relationship of two rays to each other. If the rays are traveling away from each other they are diverging from a source; how much they diverge, and at any particular plane how far away they are from their source, depends on their vergence at that plane. If the rays are traveling toward each other, they are converging toward a point; how much they converge, and how far they will travel from a particular plane until they meet, depends on their vergence at that plane. A flat reflecting surface will not change the vergence of the rays striking it, so an image seen in a mirror appears to be as far behind the mirror as the object is in front of the mirror.

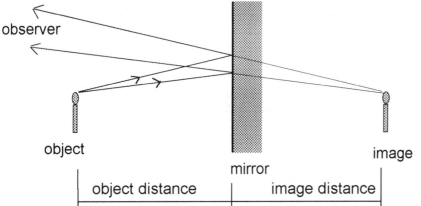

If the surface of the reflecting material is curved, then the vergence of the reflected rays will change. We can think of a spherical reflecting surface as if it were made up of a series of very small flat reflecting surfaces. If a very small light source is placed at the center of the sphere that created the curved surface, then the light rays traveling from the center to the small flat surface will be perpendicular to the surfaces, and will travel right back to the little light. (After the rays reflect from the surface and arrive back at the center of the curve, the rays continue on to the left, diverging from the light.)

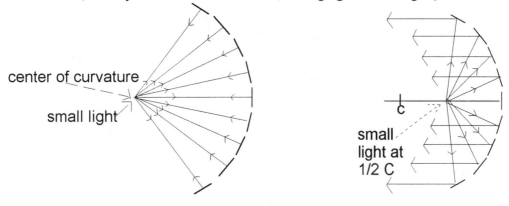

If the very small light source is placed one-half of the distance between the center of curvature and the surface of the spherical mirror, the rays will reflect back parallel to the line between the center and the light.

In each of the following diagrams the light rays are diverging from the small light source, and the spherical concave reflecting surface changes the vergence of the rays. In the case where the light source is at the center of curvature of the surface, the rays change from diverging to converging rays. They converge back toward the source (and then diverge again in the new direction). In the diagram where the light source is at 1/2 the length of the radius of the curve, the rays change from diverging to zero (or no vergence.)

A concave reflecting surface is a converging surface, just as a convex refracting surface (or lens) is a converging surface. The point from which diverging rays will be reflected parallel to each other is the focal point of the reflecting surface. Therefore, the focal length of a curved mirror is equal to one-half of the radius of curvature. When we discussed lenses we agreed to call a converging lens a plus lens, and to call its focal length a positive focal length. Therefore, a concave mirror has a positive focal length.

A convex reflecting surface, then, has a negative focal length and is a diverging surface. Incident parallel rays of light will diverge after reflection from the surface. Their vergence will be the same as it would have been if they had originated at a point called the focal point that is to the right of the convex mirror. Rays of light that are converging toward each other such that they would meet at the focal point will be reflected parallel to each other by the convex mirror.

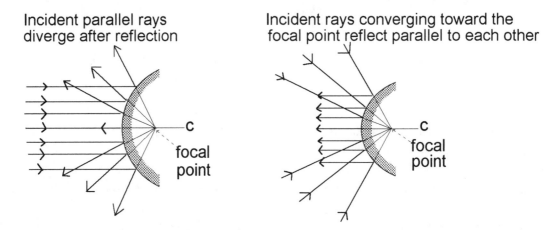

We need to define several terms. The **center of curvature,** as we have seen, is the point that is equidistant from every point of the sphere that describes the curved mirror. The **axis** of the mirror can be any ray that passes through the center of curvature. In the following discussion, we will use as the axis a ray that goes through both the object and the center of curvature. The **focal point** is the point on the axis that is 1/2 the distance from the center of curvature to the mirror. Rays of light emerging from a small light at the focal point reflect from a converging mirror parallel to the axis. The **vertex** is the point where the axis touches the mirror. Notice that for spherical mirrors, although there is only one center of curvature, there are an infinite number of axis, focal points and vertices. Once an axis is chosen, there is only one focal point and only one vertex.

Look at what happens to the light rays that bounce off of an object and travel toward a concave mirror. Rays of light bounce off every point on the object, and many travel toward the mirror:

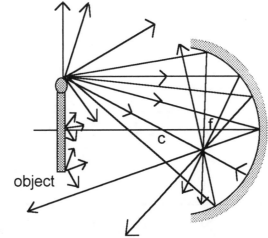

object

observer

The rays that are reflected back from the surface of the mirror will cross at some point, and continue on. The light rays will appear to an observer to be diverging from the point where they all crossed. The image appears to be at that point. When an observer looks toward the mirror, the object will appear to be where the rays crossed.

Consider several particular rays that just happen to travel in directions that allow us to follow their paths.

> 1. The ray that travels parallel to the axis is reflected so that it passes through the focal point.
> 2. The ray that travels through the focal point reflects back parallel to the axis. This statement is a definition of the focal point.
> 3. The ray that travels through the center of curvature is reflected back on itself.
> 4. The ray that touches the mirror at the vertex is reflected back at the exact same distance below the axis that it had been above the axis.

In the diagram on the next page, the particular rays that are drawn happen to be coming from the head of the object and are traveling toward the mirror. The reflected image of the head of the object that is seen by an observer *appears* to form where the rays cross and continue on. To an observer to the left of the mirror, the rays *appear* to originate at the point where they cross, since they are diverging from that point.

We need an agreement on what is negative and what is positive. We already agreed that the concave mirror has a positive focal length. We will now state that the object distance, p, is positive if it is to the left of the mirror. (For single mirrors, p is always positive. If several mirrors or lenses are lined up in a series, p may not be always positive.) For mirrors, if the image is to the left of the mirror, we will consider the image distance, q, to be positive. We will also state that if the object or the image is above the axis then its length (or the distance to the axis) will be positive. In the diagram above the *image distance q is positive*, but the distance from the axis to *the top of the image* is negative.

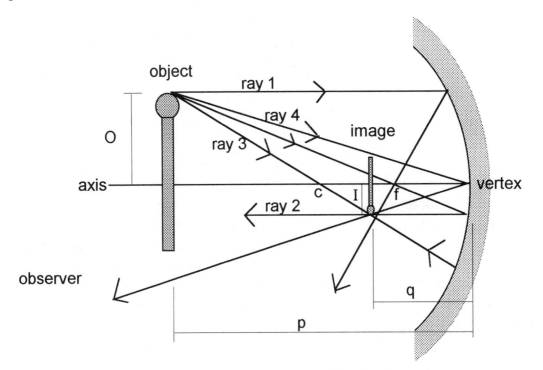

Note: Some texts use l and l' for image and object distance, some use s and s', some use u and v, and some use p and q. We will use p and q in this text. We chose to use p and q instead of l and l' or s and s' because the notation using ' is hard to see and can cause unnecessary confusion.

Using p to represent the distance from the object to the mirror, and q to represent the distance from the mirror to where the image forms, the image distance formula is

$$\frac{1}{f} = \frac{1}{p} + \frac{1}{q}, \text{ or } \frac{1}{q} = \frac{1}{f} - \frac{1}{p}$$

We will now define the object size, or the distance from the axis to the top of the object, to be O, and the image size, or the distance from the axis to the point where the top of the image *forms*, to be I. The **linear magnification,** or ratio of image size to object size, will be M.

The linear magnification is

$$M = -\frac{q}{p} = \frac{I}{O}$$

where M = linear magnification,
O = distance of the tip of the object from the axis,
I = distance of the tip of the image from the axis.

For practical purposes, use

$$I = (M)(O)$$

We will try a few examples. A good way to practice is with graph paper and colored pencils. As you do the drawings for yourself, you will notice one potentially disturbing fact: the four rays, when correctly drawn, do not cross at exactly the same point. The rule that the focal point is at 1/2 the radius of curvature is actually true only if the object size O is small with respect to the focal length of the mirror. O is not small with respect to the focal length in our drawings. This disparity in the drawings is a demonstration of **spherical aberration.** Spherical aberration means that the rays that are not **paraxial,** or close to the axis, have a shorter focal length than rays that are close to the axis. This aberration is corrected by using parabolic curves for the mirror (or for a lens), instead of spherical curves. The focal length of any spherical mirror or lens is shorter at the periphery of the lens than at its optical center.

Note: f, p, and q may be in any unit, as long as they are in the *same* unit. Likewise, I and O may be in any unit, as long as they are the same unit. They need not be the same unit as f, p, and q. M is a ratio, and has no unit.

EXAMPLE 1: A concave mirror has a focal length of 20mm. If a 24mm object is 80mm from the mirror, where does the image form? What is the size and orientation of the image?

f is 20mm
p is 80mm
O is 24mm.

Using the image distance formula,

$$\frac{1}{q} = \frac{1}{f} - \frac{1}{p}$$

$$= \frac{1}{20} - \frac{1}{80} = 0.05 - 0.0125 = 0.0375$$

Since $1/q = 0.0375$, $q = 1/0.0375 = \mathbf{27mm}$.
Using the magnification formula,

$$\mathbf{M} = -\frac{q}{p} = -\frac{27}{80} = \mathbf{-0.34}$$

so $\mathbf{I} = (M)(O) = (24)(-0.34) = \mathbf{-8mm}$.

Using a cm ruler and the diagram on page 158, you can verify both the 27mm distance for q, and the 8mm length for I. If we had not already drawn the diagram to show where the image is, we would be able to tell several facts from these numbers.

1. q is positive, so the image is to the left of the mirror.
2. M is negative, so the image is inverted from the orientation of the object.

3. I is negative, so the image is forming inverted, below the axis.
4. M is less than 1, so the image is smaller than the object. It is *minified*.

EXAMPLE 2: Suppose a concave converging mirror has a center of curvature of 50mm, and a 23mm object is placed 37mm from the vertex of the mirror surface. Where does the image form, and what is the linear magnification and the image size?

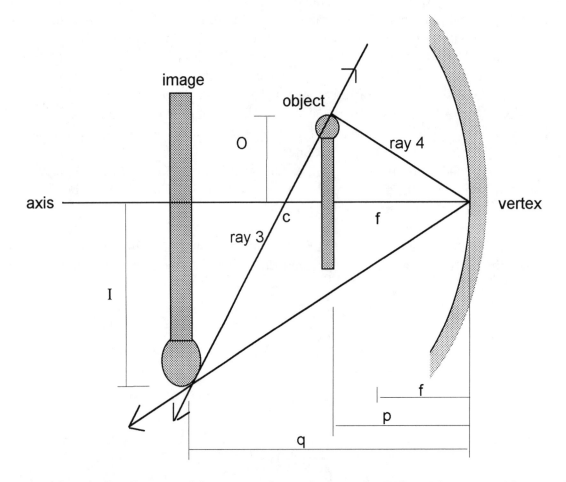

f is 1/2 the distance of the center of curvature, so f = 50/2 = 25mm. *p* = 37mm and O = 23mm.

$$\frac{1}{q} = \frac{1}{f} - \frac{1}{p}$$

$$= \frac{1}{25} - \frac{1}{37} = 0.04 - 0.0270 = 0.0130$$

Since 1/*q* = 0.0130, *q* = 1/0.0130 = **77mm**.

Using the magnification formula,

$$M = -\frac{q}{p} = -\frac{77}{37} = -2.1$$

so $I = (M)(O) = (23)(-2.1) = -48mm$.

We may now state several facts from these numbers.

1. q is positive, so the image is to the left of the mirror.
2. M is negative, so the image is inverted from the orientation of the object.
3. I is negative, so the image is forming inverted, below the axis.
4. M is greater than 1, so the image is larger than the object. It is **_magnified._**

Notice that, in both of these exercises, only rays 3 and 4 were drawn. These two rays do not depend on the rule that f is 1/2 of the radius of curvature, so they do not result in spherical aberration. We will not be so lucky when we do drawings with lenses! Draw rays 1 and 2 on the diagrams so you can see that they give image positions that are similar, but not exact, as rays 3 and 4 do.

Now we will try a convex, diverging mirror. This mirror has a negative focal length. The rays are drawn from the object so that they _would have_ gone through the center or through the focal point, _had the mirror not been there_, and then reflected according to the rules on page 157.

Spherical aberration again shows up with ray 1, which does not go where it should. Had the focal length been shorter for this ray, or had the curve of the mirror been parabolic instead of spherical, the ray would form correctly. This ray is "too far from the axis" in comparison to the focal length and radius of the sphere.

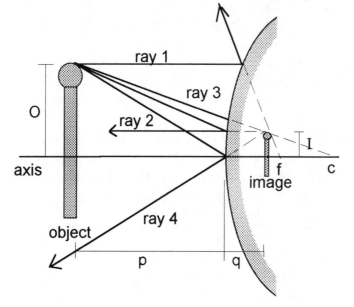

Using this drawing, the distances are $f = -15mm$, $p = 40mm$, and $O = 24mm$.

$$\frac{1}{q} = \frac{1}{f} - \frac{1}{p}$$

$$= \frac{1}{-15} - \frac{1}{40} = -0.0667 - 0.02570 = -0.0917$$

Since $1/q = -0.0917$, $q = 1/(-0.0917) = \textbf{-11mm}$.

Using the magnification formula,

$$\mathbf{M} = -\frac{q}{p} = -\frac{-11}{40} = \textbf{+0.28}$$

$$\mathbf{I} = (M)(O) = (24)(0.28) = \textbf{7mm.}$$

1. q is negative, so the image is to the right of the mirror.
2. M is positive, so the image has the same orientation to the object.
3. I is positive, so the image is forming erect, above the axis.
4. M is less than 1, so the image is smaller than the object. It is *minified*.

We are ready to state more rules of the road:

---

1. If the linear magnification, M, is positive, then the image has the same orientation as the object. If M is negative, the image has the opposite orientation from the object.
2 If the length of the image, I, is positive, the image is above the axis. If I is negative, the image is below the axis.
3. If the image distance, q, is positive, the image is to the left of the mirror. This image is ***real***. It will actually form on a piece of film placed at the plane where the rays cross.
4. If the image distance, q, is negative, the image is to the right of the mirror. This image is ***virtual***. The rays appear to diverge from there, so it appears to be present to the observer, who is to the left of the mirror. But the rays of light do not ever actually pass through the position where the image appears to form, so it cannot be formed on a piece of film at that place.
5. If the linear magnification, M, is between zero and one, then the image is smaller than the object, or ***minified***. If M is greater than one, the image is larger than the object, or ***magnified***. If M is equal to one, the image and the object are the same size. (In using this rule, use the absolute value of M; ignore the sign of M).

When there is only one imaging element, such as one mirror or one lens, then an erect image is always virtual. So both the negative M and the negative I indicate that the image is real, and a positive M and a positive I indicate that the image is virtual. However, the object for a lens or mirror could be either real or virtual when there is more than one element, such as in a telescope or in a microscope. In a multiple-element system, a negative M simply means that the image has the opposite orientation from the object. The only time the image must be virtual is when the image distance, q, is negative.

Ready to try a few? The exercises will be easier if you use graph paper. For some of the exercises, it may be easier to use the formulas first to see where the image should be forming; in others it may be easier to make the drawings first. Remember, the most accurate rays are those that do not use the focal point.

MIRROR IMAGE FORMATION EXERCISES
(Round all measurements to whole mm.)

1. Do a series of drawings, all with a concave converging mirror having a focal length of 40mm and an object size of 20mm. Use the formulas to compute q, M and I.
   a. $p = 100$mm.
   b. $p = 80$mm (where the center of curvature is).
   c. $p = 60$mm.
   d. $p = 40$mm (where the focal point is).
   e. $p = 20$mm.

   What conclusions can you make from these drawings about image formation in a converging mirror?

2. Do a series of drawings, all with a convex diverging mirror having a focal length of −40mm and an object size of 20mm. Use the formulas to compute q, M and I.
   a. $p = 80$mm.
   b. $p = 40$mm.
   c. $p = 20$mm.

   What conclusions can you make from these drawings about image formation in a diverging mirror?

3. The focal length of a plano mirror is infinity. 1/f approaches 0 as f becomes very large. Use the image placement and linear magnification formulas to demonstrate the truth of the placement of the image in the flat mirror on page 155.

4. Where does the image form, and what is its orientation, if an object is between the center of curvature and the focal point of a concave mirror? Is the image real or virtual, and is the image larger or smaller than the object?

THINK ABOUT IT:
1. There is a mirror that is normally called a magnifying mirror in most dispensaries. Demonstrate the answers you got in problem 1, by watching the image of yourself in the mirror when you are at various distances from the mirror. What is the approximate focal length of your mirror? What is the length of the radius of curvature of your mirror?
2. What kind of mirror is the left-side rear view mirror mounted on most cars? Notice that the images are smaller, but also closer than the objects; yet we interpret the images to be farther away than the actual objects are. Why?

IMAGE SIZE AND PLACEMENT: THIN LENSES
We are going to do the same things with lenses that we did with mirrors. There are a few differences from mirrors, and we are going to make a few assumptions.

1. Assume that the lens in infinitely thin. We will discuss what happens with thick lenses next.

2. Assume that all light waves have the same refractive index in a material, so that all colors have the same focal point for a given lens. (The fact that this assumption is not true results in chromatic aberrations, which was discussed very briefly in Section II.)

3. Assume that the lens has the same material on both sides. We normally think of the lenses being in air. They could just as well be in water, as long as the water is on both sides of the lens. We will look at what happens when there are different materials on each side of the lens on pages 180-184.

4. For mirrors, the ray through the center of curvature, which reflected back upon itself, has no corresponding ray when using lenses. So we have only three principal rays, and only one of them does not depend on the assumption that the rays are paraxial, or 'close' to the axis.

5. A positive image distance q, resulting in a real image, is on the right of the lens. A negative image distance q, resulting in a virtual image, is on the left of the lens.

6. For a mirror, any line passing through the center of curvature could be an axis. For lenses, the *axis* is the line that passes *through the centers of curvature of both surfaces*.

7. For now, the point where the axis passes through the lens will be called the **optical center**. The optical center takes the place of the vertex for the mirrors.

8. For a plus lens, the point on the axis where all of the rays diverging from a small source will emerge from the lens traveling parallel to the axis is the **primary focal point**.

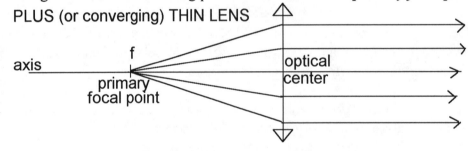

For a minus lens, the **primary focal point** is the point on the axis *toward which* rays are converging before they reach the lens, but when they emerge from the lens they are traveling parallel to the axis.

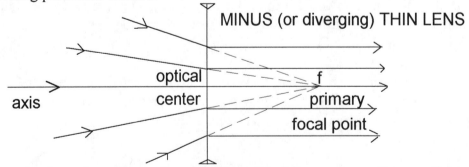

9. For a plus lens, the point on the axis where all incident rays traveling parallel to the axis cross after emerging from the lens is the **secondary focal point.** (For mirrors the primary and secondary focal points coincide.)

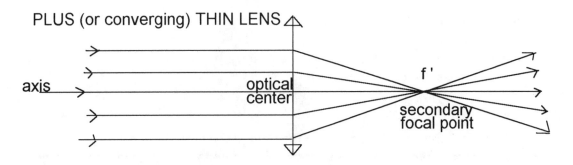

PLUS (or converging) THIN LENS

axis → optical center   f'

secondary focal point

For a minus lens, the point on the axis that all incident rays traveling parallel to the axis appear to be diverging from after emerging from the lens is the **secondary focal point**.

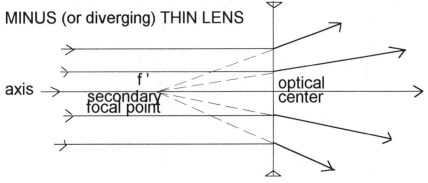

MINUS (or diverging) THIN LENS

axis →   f' secondary focal point   optical center

A plus lens will be represented by a straight line with base-in prisms at the top and bottom. A minus lens will be represented by a straight line with base-out prisms at the top and bottom.

The rules for ray tracing are now:

1. The ray that travels through the optical center is not deviated.
2. The ray that travels through (or toward) the primary focal point emerges parallel to the axis.
3. The ray that travels parallel to the axis emerges traveling toward (or from) the secondary focal point.

The formulas remain exactly the same as the mirror imaging formulas.

EXAMPLE 1: A lens with focal length of +30mm (what is its dioptric value?) has a 10mm tall object that is 50mm away. What type of image is produced, how tall is it, and where is it located?

$$\frac{1}{q} = \frac{1}{f} - \frac{1}{p} = \frac{1}{30} - \frac{1}{50} = 0.0333 - 0.02 = 0.0133$$

Since $1/q = 0.01333$, $q = 1/0.01333 =$ **75mm**.

Using the magnification formula,

$$M = -\frac{q}{p} = -\frac{75}{50} = -1.5$$

$$I = (M)(O) = (10)(-1.5) = -15mm$$

1. p is positive, so the image is to the right of the lens. It is real.
2. M is negative, so the image forms with the opposite orientation to the object.
3. I is negative, so the image is forming inverted, below the axis.
4. M is greater than 1, so the image is larger than the object. It is magnified.

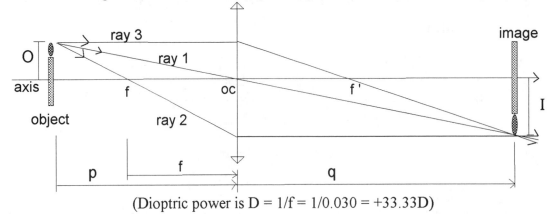

(Dioptric power is D = 1/f = 1/0.030 = +33.33D)

The next example will be a diverging lens. Remember, when drawing the rays, that they are the rays that *would have gone through a particular point* had the lens not been there. The emerging rays are diverging from each other, so we draw back to see where they *would have originated from* in order to be traveling in their observed direction. Where the rays appear to be diverging from is where the image *appears* to form. But since the rays do not actually come from this point, the image is virtual.

EXAMPLE 2: A diverging lens has a focal length of −30mm, an image size of 10mm, and an image distance of 50mm. What is the image distance and size?

$$\frac{1}{q} = \frac{1}{f} - \frac{1}{q} = \frac{1}{-30} - \frac{1}{50} = -0.0333 - 0.02 = -0.0533$$

Since $1/q = -0.05333$ $q = 1/(-0.05333) = -19mm$. Using the magnification formula,

$$M = -\frac{q}{p} = -\frac{-19}{50} = +0.38$$

$$I = (M)(O) = (10)(0.38) = 4mm$$

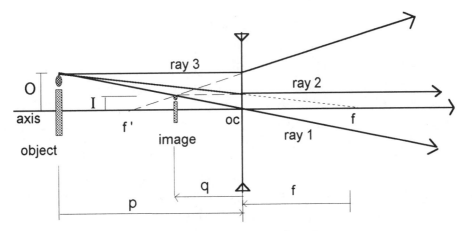

1. q is negative, so the image is to the left of the lens. It is virtual.
2. M is positive, so the image has the same orientation to the object.
3. I is positive, so the image is forming erect, above the axis.
4. M is less than 1, so the image is smaller than the object. It is minified.

THIN LENS IMAGE FORMATION EXERCISES
(Round all measurements to whole mm.)

1. Do a series of drawings, all with a convex converging thin lens having a focal length of 40mm and an object size of 20mm. Use the formulas to compute q, M, and I.
    a. $p = 100$mm.
    b. $p = 40$mm (where the primary focal point is).
    c. $p = 20$mm.
    What conclusions can you make from these drawings about image formation in a converging lens?

2. Do a series of drawings, all with a concave diverging lens having a focal length of −40mm and an object size of 20mm. Use the formulas to compute q, M, and I.
    a. $p = 80$mm.
    b. $p = 60$mm.
    c. $p = 20$mm.
    What conclusions can you make from these drawings about image formation in a diverging lens?

TRY IT: Demonstrate the answers you got in problems 1 and 2. Use a spherical lens with 3 or more diopters of plus power, and another with 3 or more diopters of minus power. Hold each lens out at a normal reading distance and watch what happens to the images of objects at various distances on the other side of the lens. What is the approximate focal length of the converging lens? If you hold the converging lens close to your eye, why are all of the images formed magnified and erect?

PRINCIPAL PLANES

When drawing the principal rays for image formation, we assumed that the thickness of the lens was not important. However, at the beginning of this section we discovered that the front and back vertex powers of a thick lens are not equal. The front vertex power is derived from the distance between the front vertex, where the optical axis enters the front surface of the lens, and the primary focal point. The back vertex power is derived from the distance between the back vertex and the secondary focal point. (see discussion on pages 151-154.)

We are going to deal only with single lenses having two spherical surfaces, made of a refracting material, and having a particular thickness. The lenses are spherical, so each surface has a center of curvature. In an earlier section we defined the radius to be *positive* for convex surfaces and *negative* for concave surfaces, which is the way most of us think of lenses in real life. Most physics and optical theory books define positive and negative radii based on whether the center of curvature is to the left (negative) or right (positive) of the lens surface. Using this definition, a bi-convex lens has a front surface radius that is positive and a back surface radius that is negative. A meniscus lens has two surfaces with positive radii. We also defined the surface power formula as $D = (n-1)/r$. It is now $D = (n_r - n_i)/r$. When a ray enters the front surface of a lens from air this formula reduces to $D_1 = (n-1)/r_1$. When the ray leaves the lens traveling back into air the formula reduces to $D_2 = (1-n)/r_2$.

The **axis of the lens** is the imaginary ray traveling through both of the centers of curvature. The **front surface** will be the surface on the left in our drawings; for meniscus lenses, the plus power surface will be the front surface. The **front vertex, V_1,** will be where the axis touches the front surface and enters the lens. The **back vertex, V_2,** will be where the axis touches the back surface and exits the lens. Aside from the radius of curvature, *for lenses positive distances* are distances where the travel is measured from left to right. All vertical measurements made above the axis will be *positive distances*. All thicknesses and radii of curvature will be in *meters*. We will assume that all rays that we trace are *paraxial,* that is, they are close to the axis. Assuming that all rays are paraxial allows us to ignore the effects of spherical lens aberrations.

As we go through the concepts and formulas below, keep in mind that there are some formulas that can be written in several forms, so you may have seen them written differently in physics books or in optical theory books. This book has the formulas in forms that are consistent with the way we use the concepts in our more basic formulas. We will use D for dioptric power and f for focal length, because these initials are what we use every day.

PRINCIPAL PLANE LOCATION IN THICK LENSES

When we diagrammed thin lenses, we constructed a single principal plane and called it the plane where all of the refraction occurred. Because we were assuming that the lens had only one focal length, using only one plane was acceptable. Since thick lenses have two focal lengths based on the lens vertices, as shown by the thick lens formulas, we will diagram the thick lens with two principal planes: P_1 and P_2. The location of the *first principal plane* is found by determining where the ray that enters the lens from the primary focal point would bend *just one time* in order to exit parallel to the axis.

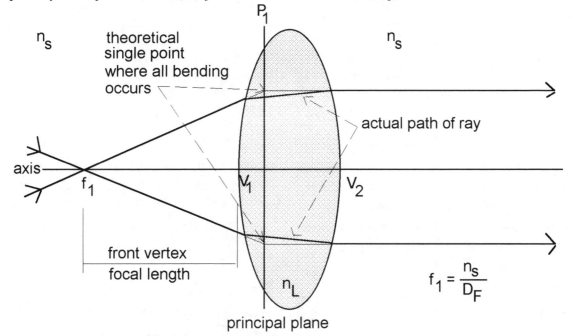

The location of the **second principal plane** is found by determining where the ray that enters the lens parallel to the axis would bend *just one time* in order to exit toward the secondary focal point.

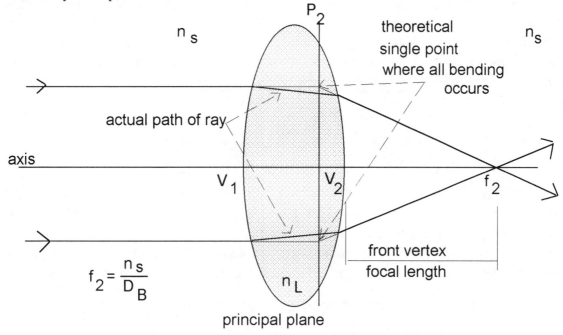

The front focal length is the distance from f_1 to V_1. The back focal length is the distance from V_2 to f_2. They are equal only if the front and back surfaces have equal curvature. The formulas for the front and back vertex powers are

$$D_B = \cfrac{D_1}{1 - (^t/n_L)\, D_1} + D_2 \qquad\qquad D_F = \cfrac{D_2}{1 - (^t/n_L)\, D_2} + D_1$$

where t is the distance between the front and back vertices in meters,

n_L is the index of refraction of the lens material.

The two focal lengths are

$$f_1 = n_s/D_F \ (= 1/D_F \text{ in air}) \qquad\qquad f_2 = n_s/D_B = (1/D_B \text{ in air}),$$

where n_s is the index of the material surrounding the lens.

Note: Physics textbooks use F instead of D in these formulas. The value being quantified is actually the **vergence** and not the dioptric value represented by the focal length f. We will continue to use D instead of F for the vergence in order to keep the notation consistent with the rest of this text.

PLUS (or converging) THIN LENS

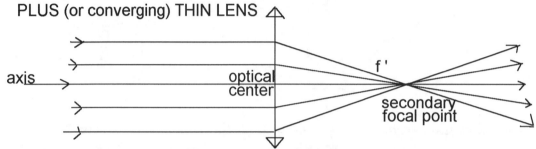

Next we need the ***equivalent power formula.*** The equivalent power has two uses. When several lenses are lined up in series, the equivalent power is the power needed for a single lens to provide the same power as the series of lenses. This definition is the more general concept. For a lens system with a single thick lens, the equivalent power formula provides the position of the principal planes *with respect to the first and second focal points*. The equivalent power formula for a single thick lens is

$$\boxed{D_{eq} = D_1 + D_2 - {}^t/_n D_1 D_2}$$

and $f = n_s/D_{eq}$ (= $1/D_{eq}$ when the lens is in air).

Using this definition of f, we can now locate the principal planes with respect to the lens vertices. H_1 and H_2 are the ***principal points***, the points where the principal planes cross the axis. f is the distance from f_1 to H_1, and also the distance from H_2 to f_2. (See the drawing on the next page.)

When we do ray tracings on thin lenses, we assume that the two principal planes coincide, and the point where that plane crosses the axis is the optical center. We will determine exactly where the optical center for a thick lens is with the formula

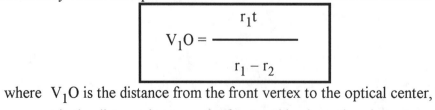

where V_1O is the distance from the front vertex to the optical center,

t is the distance between the front and back vertices in meters,

r_1 is the radius of curvature of the front surface,

r_2 is the radius of curvature of the back surface.

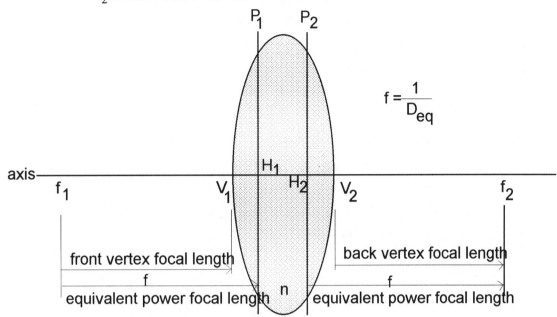

Notice that the placement of the optical center did not contain n. It is dependent solely on the curves and the thickness. The optical center is the only point that *does not disperse white light into colors*, since it is not dependent on n.

Lets analyze the principle plane positions for a few lenses before we eliminate the surfaces and use the principal planes to predict where images will form.

EXAMPLE 1: A thick lens in air made of a material with index of refraction of 1.50 has a front surface power of +15.00D, a back surface power of +5.00D, and a thickness of 32mm.

$D_1 = +15.00D$

$D_2 = +5.00D$

$n = 1.50$

$t = 32mm = 0.032m$

$r_1 = (n-1)/D_1 = 0.5/15 = +0.0333m$

$r_2 = (1-n)/D_2 = -0.5/5 = -0.1m$ *(See page 168 for the change in the formula for r.)*

$$D_B = \frac{D_1}{1-(t/n)D_1} + D_2 = \frac{+15}{1-(0.032/1.5)(15)} + 5 = \frac{15}{0.68} + 5 = 22.06 + 5$$

$D_B = +27.06D$

$f_2 = 1/D_B = 1/27.06 = 0.037m = 37mm$

$$D_F = \frac{D_2}{1-(t/n)D_2} + D_1 = \frac{+5}{1-(0.032/1.5)(5)} + 15 = \frac{5}{0.893} + 15$$

$D_F = 5.60 + 15 = \textbf{+20.60D}$

$f_1 = 1/D_F = 1/20.60 = 0.049m = \textbf{49mm}$

$D_{eq} = D_1 + D_2 - (t/n)D_1D_2 = +15 +5 - (0.032/1.5)(15)(5)$

$D_{eq} = 20 - 1.6 = \textbf{+18.40D}$

$f = 1/D_{eq} = 1/18.40 = 0.054m = \textbf{54mm}$

$V_1O = (r_1 t)/(r_1 - r_2) = (0.033)(0.032)/(0.033 + 0.1)$

$V_1O = (0.00106)/(0.133) = 0.008m = \textbf{8mm}$

Notice on the drawing that the principal planes have shifted toward the surface with the steeper curve, as has the optical center.

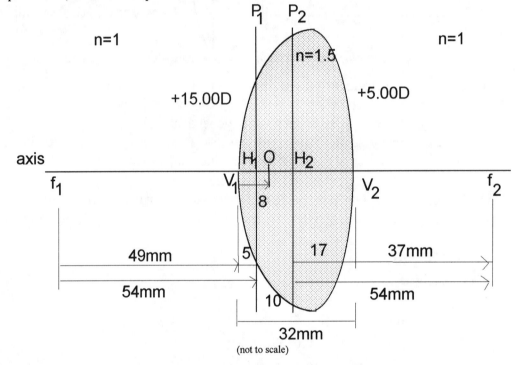

(not to scale)

EXAMPLE 2: A meniscus thick lens made of flint glass, n = 1.70, has a front surface power of +20.00D, a back surface power of −5.00D, and a thickness of 19mm.

$D_1 = \textbf{+20}$

$D_2 = \textbf{−5}$

$n = \textbf{1.70}$

$t = 19mm = \textbf{0.019m}$

$r_1 = (n-1)/D_1 = 0.7/20 = \textbf{+0.035m}$

$r_2 = (1-n)/D_2 = -0.7/(-5) = \textbf{+0.14m}$

$$D_B = \frac{D_1}{1 - (t/n)D_1} + D_2 = \frac{+20}{1 - (0.019/1.7)(20)} - 5 = \frac{20}{0.776} - 5$$

$\mathbf{D_B} = 25.76 - 5 = \mathbf{+20.76D}$

$\mathbf{f_2} = 1/D_B = 1/20.76 = 0.048m = \mathbf{48mm}$

$$D_F = \frac{D_2}{1 - (t/n)D_2} + D_1 = \frac{-5}{1 - (0.019/1.7)(-5)} + 20 = \frac{-5}{1.056} + 20$$

$\mathbf{D_F} = -4.74 + 20 = \mathbf{+15.26D}$

$\mathbf{f_1} = 1/D_F = 1/15.26 = 0.066m = \mathbf{66mm}$

$D_{eq} = D_1 + D_2 - (t/n)D_1 D_2 = +20 - 5 - (0.019/1.7)(20)(-5)$

$\mathbf{D_{eq}} = 15 + 1.12 = \mathbf{+16.12D}$

$\mathbf{f} = 1/D_{eq} = 1/16.12 = 0.062m = \mathbf{62mm}$

$V_1 O = (r_1 t)/(r_1 - r_2) = (0.035)(0.019)/(0.035 - 0.14)$

$\mathbf{V_1 O} = (0.00067)/(-0.105) = -0.0063m = \mathbf{-6mm}$

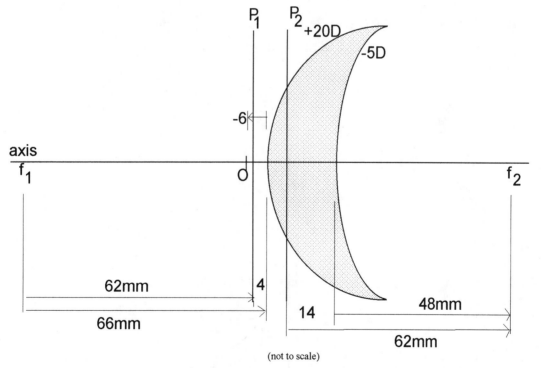

(not to scale)

Now the principal planes have shifted even further toward the steeper curve, and not only is the optical center outside of the lens, it is not even between the principal planes!

EXAMPLE 3: A meniscus thick lens made of polycarbonate, n = 1.586, has a front
surface power of +2.00D, a back surface power of –25.00D, and a thickness of 5mm.

$D_1 = +2$

$D_2 = -25$

$n = 1.586$

$t = 5mm = 0.005m$

$r_1 = (n-1)/D_1 = 0.586/2 = +0.293m$

$r_2 = (1-n)/D_2 = -0.586/(-25) = +0.023m$

$$D_B = \frac{D_1}{1-(t/n)D_1} + D_2 = \frac{+2}{1-(0.005/1.586)(2)} - 25 = \frac{2}{0.994} - 25$$

$D_B = 2.01 - 25 = -22.99D$

$f_2 = 1/D_B = 1/22.99 = -0.044m = -44mm$

$$D_F = \frac{D_2}{1-(t/n)D_2} + D_1 = \frac{-25}{1-(0.005/1.586)(-25)} + 2 = \frac{-25}{1.079} + 2$$

$D_F = -23.17 + 2 = -21.17D$

$f_1 = 1/D_F = 1/21.17 = 0.047m = -47mm$

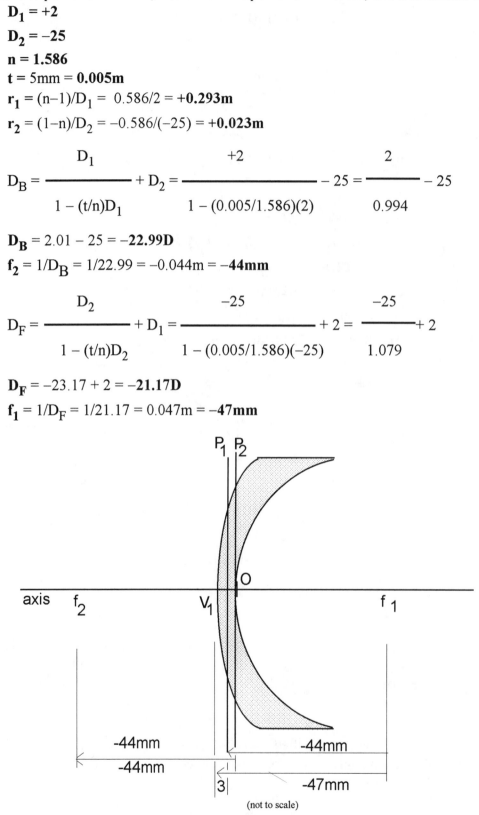

(not to scale)

$D_{eq} = D_1 + D_2 - (t/n)D_1D_2 = +2 - 25 - (0.005/1.586)(2)(-25)$

$\mathbf{D_{eq}} = -23 + 0.16 = \mathbf{-22.84D}$

$\mathbf{f} = 1/D_{eq} = 1/22.84 = -0.044m = \mathbf{-44mm}$

$V_1O = (r_1t)/(r_1 - r_2) = (0.293)(0.005)/(0.293 - 0.023)$

$\mathbf{V_1O} = (0.00147)/(0.27) = 0.0054m = \mathbf{5mm}$

The steeper side is to the back of the lens, so the principal planes and the optical center moved toward the back. Occasionally P_1 and P_2 will change sides for a minus lens; usually they remain in this order.

PRINCIPAL PLANE LOCATION EXERCISES
(Round all measurements to mm.)

1. Locate the principal planes and the optical center for a bi-convex lens made of index 1.50 plastic, if the front surface has a surface power of +35D, the back has a surface power of +1D, and the thickness at the vertices is 35mm.

2. Locate the principal planes and the optical center for a meniscus lens made of index 1.50 plastic, if the front surface has a radius of curvature of +20mm and the back surface has a radius of curvature of -50mm, and the vertices are 50mm apart.

IMAGE SIZE AND PLACEMENT: THICK LENSES

Now that we can find the position of the principal planes for any lens, we can determine where the image forms for any thick lens. The rules for ray tracing differ from the thin lens in only one way. All rays are drawn parallel to the axis as they travel from P_1 to P_2. Otherwise, the rules are the same.

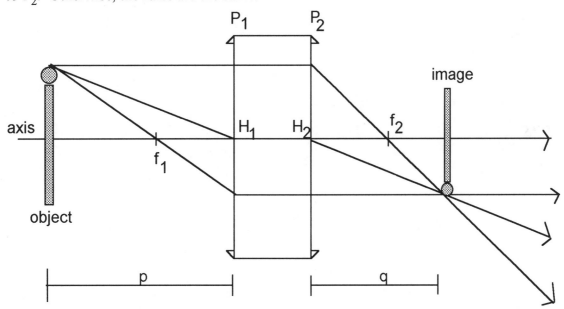

1. The ray that travels through the first principal point (H_1) emerges from the second principal point (H_2) traveling in the same direction as before. It is displaced, but it is not deviated.
2. The ray that travels through (or toward) the primary focal point bends at the first principal plane (P_1) and emerges parallel to the axis.
3. The ray that travels parallel to the axis is bent at the second principal plane (P_2) and emerges traveling toward (or from) the secondary focal point.

Keep in mind as we go through the drawings that we are not showing the actual path of the ray as it traverses the lens. We are showing the exact path of the ray *before it enters* the lens and *after it exits* the lens. What happens between the vertices and the principal planes is *constructed* so that we can explain mathematically the result of the refractions that occur at the two surfaces.

The thick minus lens, with P_1 to the left of P_2:

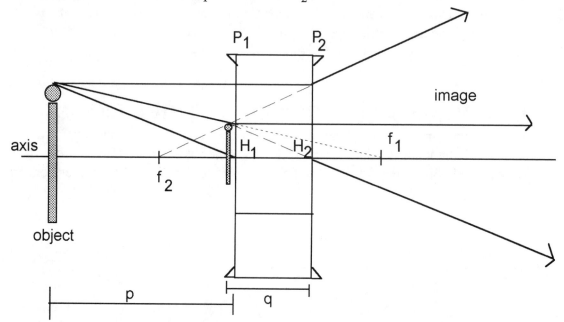

For the occasional thick minus lens where P_1 is on the right of P_2 the rays go to P_1 first, *go back to P_2 parallel to the axis*, and emerge in the correct direction from P_2.

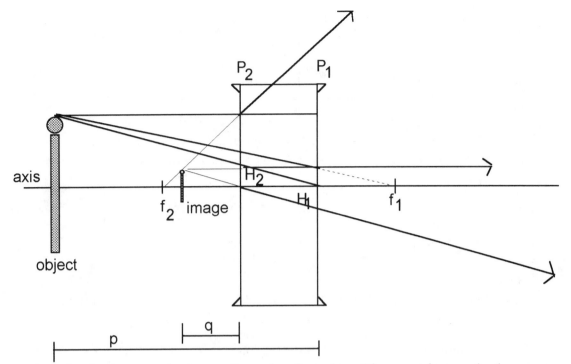

And that leads us to the image formation formulas. They remain exactly the same as for the thin lens and for the mirror. The object distance p is measured from the object to P_1, and the image distance q is measured from P_2 to the image. The focal length f is derived from the equivalent power D_{eq}. Look at the definition of D_{eq} again. It is the power needed to give the observed results using only a single thin lens. The equivalent power and the principal planes are fabricated. We create imaginary planes so that we can use formulas and ray tracings to predict the size and position of the image formed.

EXAMPLE 1 from page 171-172 is a lens with $D_1 = +15D$, $D_2 = +5D$, and f = 54mm. If an object is placed 100mm to the left of the front vertex, where does the image form, and what is the magnification?

For this lens, f_1 is 49mm to the left of the front vertex, and f is 54mm. Therefore, P_1 is 5mm to the right of the front vertex, and the object distance p, which is measured to P_1, is 105mm.

Using the image formation formula,

$$\frac{1}{q} = \frac{1}{f} - \frac{1}{p} = \frac{1}{54} - \frac{1}{105} = 0.0185 - 0.0095 = 0.0090$$

Since $1/q = 0.009$, $q = 1/0.009 =$ **111mm**.

Using the magnification formula,

$$M = -\frac{q}{p} = -\frac{111}{105} = -1.06 = -\textbf{1.1}$$

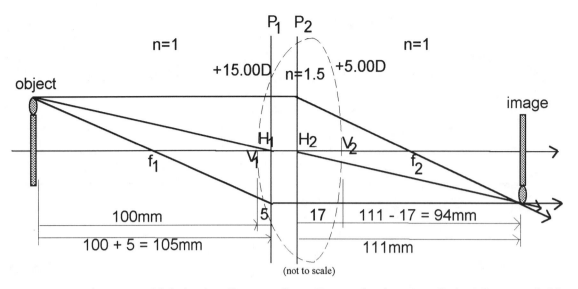

P₁ P₂

n=1

+15.00D   n=1.5   +5.00D

n=1

object

image

H₁ H₂   V₂

f₁   V₁   f₂

100mm   5   17   111 - 17 = 94mm

100 + 5 = 105mm   111mm

(not to scale)

q is 111, which is the distance from P_2 to the image. f_2 is 37mm and f is 54mm, so P_2 is 17mm to the left of the back vertex. Therefore, the image will form 111–17 = **94mm to the right of the back vertex V_2**.

1. q is positive, so the image is to the right of the lens. The image is real.
2. M is negative, so the image has the opposite orientation from the object.
3. I (not computed) would be negative for a real, or positive, object, so the image is forming inverted, below the axis.
4. M is bigger than one, so the image is magnified.

A good way to deal with each of these exercises is to get some graph paper and draw out the whole system to scale. Trace the rays, and verify for yourself that the formulas give the correct answer. Remember, the rays will only give you the approximate location and size, since the drawings violate the paraxial rule for spherical lenses. The rays that are not close to the axis show spherical aberration.

EXAMPLE 2: Look at the negative lens in example 3 on pages 174-175. For this lens f = –44mm. Where will the image be located if an object is placed 50mm from the front surface? What is the magnification for this image?

f_1 is –47mm and f is –44mm, so P_1 is 3mm to the right of the front vertex. The object distance, q, is 50 + 3 = 53mm from P_1.

$$\frac{1}{q} = \frac{1}{f} - \frac{1}{p} = \frac{1}{-44} - \frac{1}{53} = -0.023 - 0.019 = -0.042$$

Since $1/q = -0.042$, $q = 1/(-0.042) = $ **–24mm**, or the image forms 24mm to the left of P_2, which is coincident with the back vertex V_2. Using the magnification formula,

$$\mathbf{M} = -\frac{q}{p} = -\frac{-24}{53} = \mathbf{+0.5}$$

1. q is negative, so the image is to the left of the lens. The image is virtual.

2. M is positive, so the image is in the same orientation to the object.
3. I will be positive for a real, or positive, object, so the image will form above the axis.
4. M is less than 1, so the image is smaller than the object, or minified.

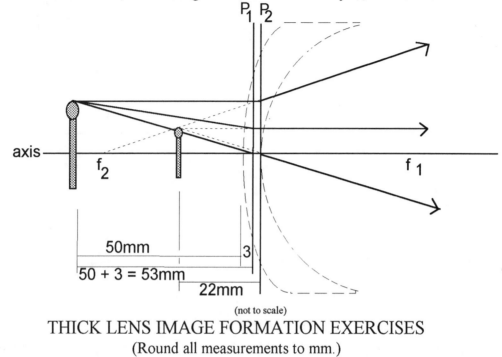

(not to scale)

THICK LENS IMAGE FORMATION EXERCISES
(Round all measurements to mm.)

1. Using the lens designed in exercise 1 on page 175, having surface powers of +35D and +1D, made of 1.50 plastic, and with a thickness at the vertices of 35mm, compute the image placement and size for a 15mm object placed:
   a. 60mm from the front vertex.
   b. 28mm from the front vertex.
   c. 15mm from the front vertex.

   Make drawings to help you conceptualize where the images are forming.

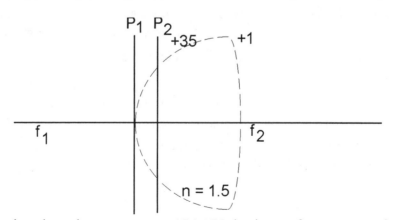

2. Using the minus lens shown on pages 174-175, having surface powers of +2D, −25D, thickness of 5mm and index 1.586, compute the image placement and size for a 15mm object placed:

a. 57mm from the front vertex.

b. 27mm from the front vertex.

Make drawings to help you conceptualize where the images are forming.

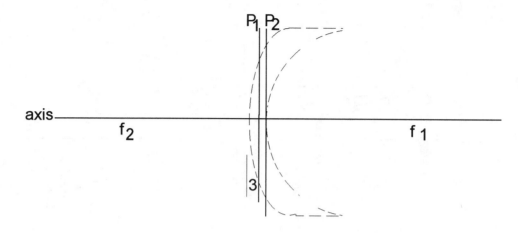

NODAL POINTS

We have one assumption left to explore. In all of our ray tracings the lenses have been surrounded by air. Immersing the lens in water or some other medium with index of refraction n_i would only affect the computations of focal length from surface powers, and surface power from radius of curvature. Go back to page 30 and page 35 in Section III to see how to adjust these computations.

What if the lens is separating two different materials? A prescription diver's mask would have air on one side and water on the other side. The eye has air on one side and vitreous on the other. Many lenses in optical instruments are composed of two or more different materials sandwiched together. Look at the path of a light ray when it enters the eye. There are several different refractions, separating a variety of media. Consider a lens made of a material with index of refraction of n_2, separating two other media with indices of n_1 (on the left) and n_3 (on the right). The index of refraction of the lens, n_2, is higher than either n_1 or n_3.

In the last several pages we have discussed the principal planes and briefly mentioned H_1 and H_2, where the principal planes cross the axis. H_1 and H_2 are called the *principal points*. When $n_1 = n_3$, the principal points are the points where the incident light ray exits the lens displaced but not deviated.

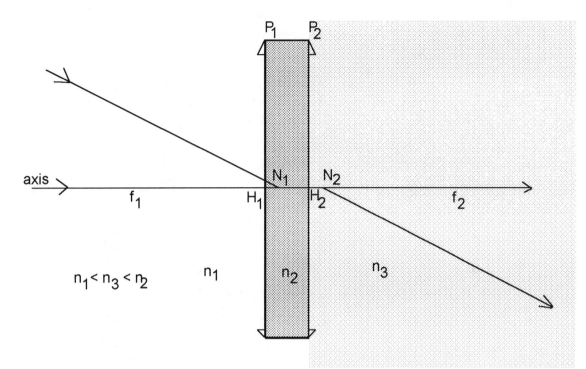

When n_1 and n_3 are not equal, the points where the incident light ray exits displaced but not deviated are the **nodal points** N_1 and N_2. The nodal points coincide with the principal points when $n_1 = n_3$. For a plus thick lens the nodal points move away from H_1 and H_2 toward the side of the lens where the denser material is; if $n_3 > n_1$, the nodal points move to the right on the diagram. For a minus thick lens the nodal points move away from H_1 and H_2 toward the side of the lens where the rarer material is; if $n_3 > n_1$, the nodal points move to the left on the diagram. The two nodal points move equal amounts: the distance from H_1 to N_1 is equal to the distance from H_2 to N_2. The distance HN that the nodal points move from the principal points is equal to

$$\boxed{HN = H_2 f_2 - f_1 H_1}$$

The **cardinal points** for a lens are the focal points, the nodal points, and the principal points.

EXAMPLE 1: A bi-convex lens made of a material with $n = 1.5$ separates air, $n = 1$, from water, $n = 1.33$, and has a center thickness of 30mm. The radius of curvature of the surface in contact with air is 25mm. The radius of curvature of the surface in contact with water is -25mm. An 11mm object is placed 50mm from the front lens surface on the side where the air is. Find the positions of all six cardinal points and the image size, orientation, and location. Verify all results with a drawing.

$n_1 = 1.0$

$n_2 = 1.5$

$n_3 = 1.33$

$r_1 = 25$mm $= 0.025$m

$D_1 = (n_2 - n_1)/r_1 = 0.5/0.025 = \mathbf{+20D}$

$r_2 = -25mm = \mathbf{-0.025m}$

$D_2 = (n_3 - n_2)/r_2 = -0.17/-0.025 = \mathbf{+6.80D}$

$t = 30mm = \mathbf{0.030m}$

$$D_B = \frac{D_1}{1 - (t/n_2)D_1} + D_2 = \frac{20}{1 - (0.030/1.5)20} + 6.80 = \frac{20}{0.6} + 6.80$$

$\mathbf{D_B} = 33.33 + 6.80 = \mathbf{+40.13D}$

$\mathbf{V_2 f_2} = n_3/D_B = 1.33/40.13 = 0.033m = \mathbf{33mm}$

$$D_F = \frac{D_2}{1 - (t/n_2)D_2} + D_1 = \frac{6.8}{1 - (0.030/1.5)6.8} + 20 = \frac{6.8}{0.864} + 20$$

$\mathbf{D_F} = 7.87 + 20 = \mathbf{+27.87D}$

$\mathbf{f_1 V_1} = n_1/D_F = 1/27.87 = 0.036m = \mathbf{36mm}$

$D_{eq} = D_1 + D_2 - (t/n_2)D_1D_2 = 20 + 6.80 - (0.030/1.5)(20)(6.80)$

$\mathbf{D_{eq}} = 26.80 - 2.72 = \mathbf{24.08D}$

$\mathbf{f_1 H_1} = n_1/D_{eq} = 1/24.08 = 0.042m = \mathbf{42mm}$

$\mathbf{H_2 f_2} = n_3/D_{eq} = 1.33/24.08 = 0.055m = \mathbf{55mm}$

$\mathbf{H_1 N_1 = H_2 N_2} = H_2 f_2 - f_1 H_1 = 55 - 42 = \mathbf{13mm}$

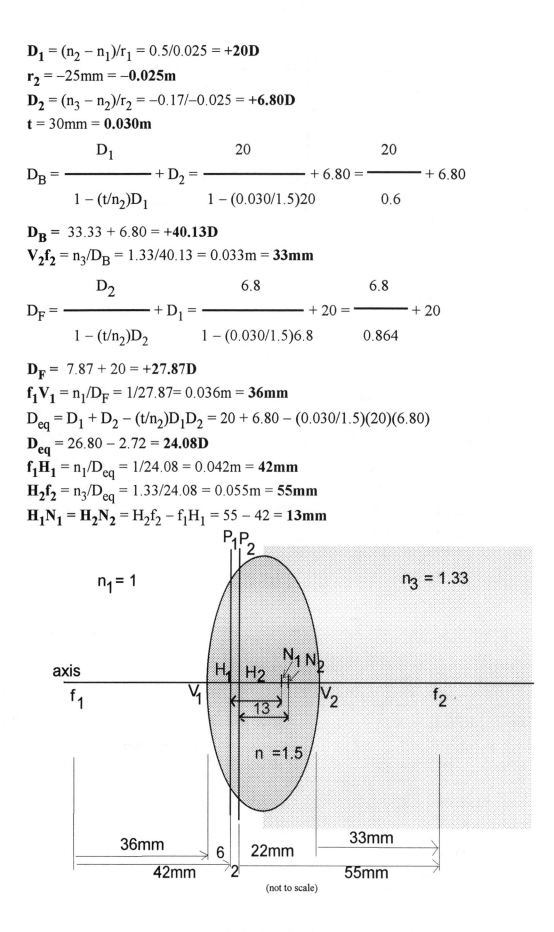

(not to scale)

Our image size and placement formulas will change slightly: p and q are to be measured *from the nodal points*, and the formula relating p and q becomes

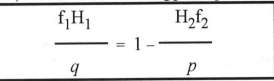

$$\frac{f_1 H_1}{q} = 1 - \frac{H_2 f_2}{p}$$

Look at the drawing to see that

p = image distance to V_1 + distance from V_1 to H_1 + distance from H_1 to N_1

$\quad = 50 + 6 + 13 = $ **69mm**

$f_1 H_1 = 42$

$H_2 f_2 = 55$

$$\frac{f_1 H_1}{q} = 1 - \frac{H_2 f_2}{p}; \qquad \frac{42}{q} = 1 - \frac{55}{69} = 1 - 0.80 = 0.20;$$

$q = 42 / 0.20 = $ **210mm**

$\mathbf{M} = -q/p = -210/69 = \mathbf{-3.0}$

$\mathbf{I} = (M)(O) = (-3.0)(11) = \mathbf{-33m}.$

q is measured to N_2. Again look at the drawing to see that V_2 to image is $210 + 13 - 22 = 201$mm; the **image is located 201mm inside the water, is real and inverted, and is 33mm long**.

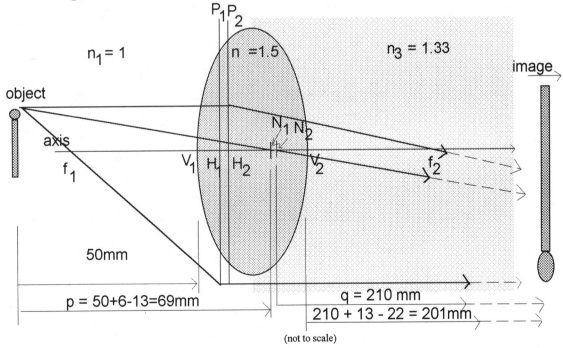

(not to scale)

NODAL POINT EXERCISE
(Round all measurements to whole mm.)

A thick lens made of flint glass, $n_2 = 1.70$, separates air, $n_1 = 1$, from plastic, $n_3 = 1.50$.

The lens has a maximum thickness of 20mm, the surface facing air has a radius of curvature of 17.5mm, and the surface facing plastic is plano. A 20mm object is placed 50mm from the front vertex of the lens. Where does the image form and what is its size?

DIAGRAM OF THE HUMAN EYE

Finally examine the human eye. Made up of several different refracting surfaces and indices, the eye can be considered as a complex system of lenses with $n_1 = 1$, $n_2 = 1.37$, $n_3 = 1.33$, $n_4 = 1.42$ and $n_5 = 1.33$, or as one optical lens consisting of the cornea and crystalline lens. In either case, there is one set of principal planes and nodal points that can be used to mathematically model what happens to the rays of light that enter the eye. The measurements in the drawing are based on Helmholtz's schematic eye. This diagram is for the emmetropic eye with no accommodation.

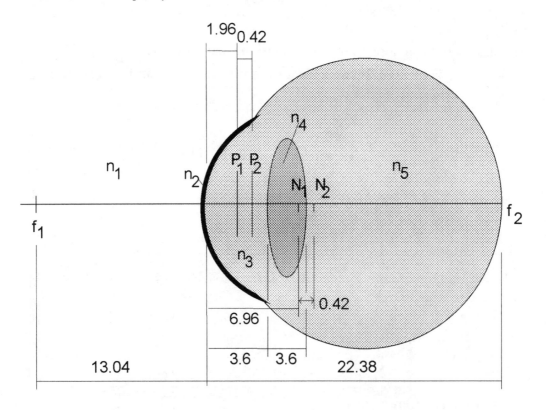

Location of principal planes and nodal points in the schematic eye.
Not to scale. All measurements in mm.
Redrawn from Pedrotti & Pedrotti, *INTRODUCTION TO OPTICS*, page 154.
H. V. Helmholtz's schematic eye 1, modified by L. Laurance.

Appendix 1
BASIC GLOSSARY

A MEASUREMENT is the distance from lens edge to lens edge, measured horizontally.

ABBE NUMBER is a measurement of the ability of a material to disperse white light into its component colors; also called Nu value, or v. It is also the inverse of relative dispersion, δ.

ABERRATIONS are properties of the lens material or lens design which result in distorted or blurred images.

ABSORPTION is the conversion of one form of energy into a different form of energy. Generally, light is absorbed as heat, although it may result in a chemical or electrical reaction.

AMBLYOPIA is a condition where the eye does not have good correctable vision, but there is no physical anomaly present in the eye.

AMETROPIA is a condition where the eye has a refractive error.

ANGLE OF INCIDENCE is the angle between a ray of light incident on a surface and the normal (or perpendicular line) to the surface at the point of incidence.

ANISOMETROPIA is an unequal refractive condition between a person's two eyes. The person is considered ANISOMETROPIC.

ASTHENOPIA is a general feeling of discomfort in or around the eyes, or a general discomfort as a result of conditions in or around the eyes.

ASTIGMATIC INTERVAL is the distance between the two focal lengths of a toric or astigmatic lens or system.

ASTIGMATISM means literally "not a point focus." Usually refers to two line foci for a single lens.

Regular astigmatism: The focal lines are at right angles to each other.

Irregular astigmatism: The focal lines are not at right angles to each other. Irregular astigmatism is usually the result of injury or disease.

With the rule astigmatism The shortest of the two focal lengths is vertical, and the correcting lens has the axis of the minus cylinder within 30° of the 0-180 meridian. When the vertical meridian of the cornea or crystalline lens is steeper than the horizontal meridian, with the rule astigmatism is the result.

Against the rule astigmatism The shortest of the two focal lengths is horizontal, and the correcting lens has the axis of the minus cylinder within 30° of the 090 meridian. When the horizontal meridian of the cornea or crystalline lens is steeper than the vertical meridian, against the rule astigmatism is the result.

Oblique astigmatism The two focal lines are between 31 and 59 degree meridian, and between 121 and 149 degree meridian.

AXIS *of a lens* is the ray that passes through the centers of curvature of both surfaces.

The *axis of a curved mirror* is any ray which travels through the center of curvature of the mirror. There are an infinite number of potential axes for a curved mirror.

The *axis of a cylinder* is the meridian of plano power or no power.

The *axis of a prescription* is the meridian on the lens where there is no cylinder power; it is the direction of the sphere power alone.

B MEASUREMENT   is the distance from lens edge to lens edge, measured vertically.

BACK FOCAL LENGTH   is the distance from the back surface vertex of a lens to the secondary focal point.

BACK VERTEX POWER   is the inverse of the back focal length in meters; it is a measurement of the ability of the lens to converge or diverge light rays. This is the power that the wearer sees and is what is measured in the focimeter or lensometer.

BOXING SYSTEM   is a system for standardizing lens and frame measurements. All measurements are in mm. This system begins by drawing a box around the lens(es) and determining the geometrical center of the lens.

CARDINAL POINTS   are the primary and secondary focal points, the principal points (where the principal planes intersect with the optical axis), and the nodal points. On a single thin lens the principal points and the nodal points coincide at the optical center of the lens.

CHROMATIC ABERRATION   is the result of the fact that light waves of different frequencies are slowed different amounts by a material. Only in a vacuum do all frequencies of the electromagnetic spectrum travel at the same speed. This property of lens materials results in images of different colors forming on different planes, resulting in slight blurring of images containing more than one frequency of light.

CIRCLE OF LEAST CONFUSION   is the plane where an astigmatic or toric lens will show the least distortion. Its distance from the lens is the inverse of the spherical equivalent of the toric lens.

COMA   is a lens aberration which results from wide beams of light traveling obliquely through a lens. It results in an elongated, blurred image. In the eye it is generally limited by the iris.

CONCAVE   1. A hollow surface; 2. A surface with negative power; 3. A lens with negative power; 4. A diverging refracting element; and 5. A converging reflecting surface.

CONSTRUCTIVE INTERFERENCE   occurs when two waves are in phase with each other, and therefore compound each other.

CONVERGENCE   is a measurement of the relative direction of travel of two light rays that are traveling toward each other. The amount of convergence of two rays at a particular plane indicates the distance the rays would have to travel from that plane in order to cross paths. Also called POSITIVE VERGENCE.

CONVEX   1. A bulging surface; 2. A surface with positive power; 3. A lens with positive power; 4. A converging refracting element; and 5. A diverging reflecting surface.

CURVATURE OF FIELD, also called CURVATURE OF IMAGE,   is a lens aberration resulting from the fact that the focal plane of a lens is curved, not flat. Most corrected curve lens designs strive to reduce or eliminate this aberration.

CYLINDER   is a surface or lens with no curvature or power in the meridian called the axis, and either positive or negative curvature or power in the meridian 90 degrees from the axis.

D MEASUREMENT   is the horizontal measurement of a lens at its midpoint. It is part of the DATUM SYSTEM of frame and lens measurement.

DATUM LINE   is the same as D MEASUREMENT.

DBL   is the distance between lenses.

DESTRUCTIVE INTERFERENCE   occurs when two waves are out of phase with each other, and therefore cancel each other.

DEVIATION   is a change of direction.

DIFFRACTION   is the bending of a wave of light when it passes through a very narrow slit or past the edge of an opaque object.

DIFFUSION   is the scattering of light rays by an irregular surface or a non-homogeneous material.

DIOPTER   is a measurement of vergence, or a measurement of the ability of a lens, prism, or mirror to change the direction of travel of incident light rays.

DIPLOPIA   is double vision.

DISPERSION   is the breaking of light into its component colors. A material's ability to disperse light is related to the different speeds of various wavelengths of visible light in the material. For some materials, like crown glass, dispersion is minimal. Other materials, like flint glass, have a larger dispersive ability.

DISPLACED   means moved or shifted to another position. For a ray of light, displaced means that it emerges in a different position from where it entered, but it may continue to travel in the original direction.

DISTORTION   is a lens aberration resulting from the increasing amounts of prism present as gaze is directed away from the optical center of a lens. This aberration is the only one of the major aberrations which does not result in a blurring of the image.

  Barrel distortion is seen in minus power lenses. Base out prism amount increases as the line of gaze travels away from the center of the lens, resulting in straight lines appearing to be concave toward the center of the lens.

  Pincushion distortion is seen in plus power lenses. Base in prism amount increases as the line of gaze travels away from the center of the lens, resulting in straight lines appearing to be convex toward the center of the lens.

DIVERGENCE   is a measurement of the relative direction of travel of two light rays that are traveling away from each other. The amount of divergence of two rays at a given plane indicates the distance the rays have traveled from their source, or since they crossed paths. Also called NEGATIVE VERGENCE.

ED or EFFECTIVE DIAMETER   is twice the longest radius of a lens measured from the geometrical center of the lens to the farthest point on the lens edge.

EMMETROPIA   is a condition of the eye where parallel incident rays of light come to a point focus on the retina when the eye is not accommodating. Needs no corrective lenses for distance vision.

EQUIVALENT POWER   of a thick lens is the power of a single infinitely thin lens needed to provide the same convergence or divergence supplied by the thick lens. This concept is used to find the locations of the principal planes.

FOCAL POINT: see PRIMARY FOCAL POINT or SECONDARY FOCAL POINT.

FOCIMETER   is an instrument used to measure the back focal length of a lens. This is the generic term, originally lensmeter. LENSOMETER and VERTOMETER are trade names.

FREQUENCY is the number of occurrences in a unit of time. For light, it is the number of waves of light that pass a particular point in one second. Measured in hertz, Hz.

FRONT FOCAL LENGTH is the distance from the front surface vertex to the primary focal point.

GEOMETRICAL CENTER of a lens is the midpoint of the horizontal and vertical measurements of the lens. This point is determined using the boxing system.

ILLUMINATION is the intensity of visible light incident on the surface of an object.

INCIDENCE: see ANGLE OF INCIDENCE.

INCIDENT SIDE is the side the light is traveling from; used when discussing the change in direction or speed of a wave of light or a photon as it travels from one material to another.

INDEX OF REFRACTION of a material, usually represented by n or μ, is the ratio of the speed of light in a vacuum to the speed of yellow light (588nm) in the material.

INTERFERENCE occurs when two waves with the same frequency either cancel or compound each other. See CONSTRUCTIVE INTERFERENCE and DESTRUCTIVE INTERFERENCE

INTERVAL OF STURM for a *toric lens* or for an *astigmatic eye* is the distance between the two focal planes.

LENSOMETER: see FOCIMETER.

LONGITUDINAL WAVE MOTION occurs when the individual particles in the supporting material travel parallel to the direction of the propagation of the wave.

LUMINOSITY is the ability of an object to emit photons or waves of light.

MARGINAL ASTIGMATISM, also called OBLIQUE ASTIGMATISM or RADIAL ASTIGMATISM, is a lens aberration resulting from the fact that waves with a horizontal orientation will have a different focal length than waves with a vertical orientation when they enter a spherical lens obliquely (not perpendicular to the surface of the lens). This aberration results in a lens inducing unwanted cylinder power when the wearer looks through the lens at an angle. See the section on Martin's Formula for Tilt, pages 128-130. Corrected curve design lenses attempt to reduce or eliminate this aberration.

MERIDIAN of a lens is any straight line on the surface of the lens, going through the optical center of the lens.

n: see INDEX OF REFRACTION.

NEGATIVE VERGENCE: see DIVERGENCE.

OBLIQUE ASTIGMATISM: see MARGINAL ASTIGMATISM.

OD refers to the right eye. It is Latin, oculus dexter.

OPACITY is a measurement of the ability of a material to absorb or reflect visible light.

OPTICAL CENTER (OC) of a lens is the point on the optical axis where any ray of light incident on the lens passes through the lens undeviated (but possibly displaced). It may be in the lens or on a surface of the lens, or it may be outside of the lens altogether.

In common usage on the thin lens the OC is the thickest part of a plus lens or the thinnest part of a minus lens; or the point on a lens surface where there is no prism power.

OPTICAL INFINITY is 20 feet or more, or 6 meters or more. Rays or waves of light that *originate* 20 feet or 6 meters or more from the observer are considered to be traveling parallel to each other when they reach the observer.

OS refers to the left eye. It is Latin, oculus sinister.

OU refers to both eyes. It is Latin, oculus uterque or oculus uniti.

P MEASUREMENT or PATTERN MEASUREMENT is the difference between the A measurement and the B measurement on a lens. The closer a lens is to square or circular, the smaller the P measurement is.

PARALLEL RAYS are rays of light which will never meet when extended in either direction. In optics, rays of light that are coming from an object 6 or more meters away are considered to be travelling parallel. This is optical infinity.

PARAXIAL rays are rays that are traveling close to the axis of a lens or mirror.

PATTERN MEASUREMENT: see P MEASUREMENT.

PD is the distance in millimeters between the visual axis of the person's eyes; generally near the center of the pupil.

PENCIL refers to a group of rays diverging from or converging on a single point of 0 dimension.

PHOTON is the basic particle of the electromagnetic spectrum. Used in quantum physics to describe some of the properties of the electromagnetic spectrum.

PLANO refers to a surface which is flat or has no curvature, or a lens with no refractive power.

POLARIZED LIGHT is light in which all of the light waves are oscillating in only one plane. This is LINEAR POLARIZATION or PLANE POLARIZATION. (Linear is preferred.) PARTIAL POLARIZATION is when the oscillations are not completely confined to one plane.

POSITIVE VERGENCE: see CONVERGENCE.

PRIMARY FOCAL POINT for a *converging lens or mirror* is the point on the optical axis from which diverging light rays will be refracted or reflected parallel to the axis as a result of the lens or mirror. For a *diverging lens or mirror*, it is the point on the optical axis toward which light rays will be converging in order for them to be refracted or reflected parallel to the axis.

PRINCIPAL PLANES are imaginary planes which can be used to describe the refraction occurring within a lens. Their positions with respect to the front and/or back vertices of a lens can be determined using the FRONT and BACK VERTEX POWER FORMULAS and the EQUIVALENT POWER FORMULA.

PRINCIPAL POINTS are the points where the principal planes cross the axis of the lens.

RAY refers to the path of a single photon of light.

REAL IMAGE is an image which results from converging rays. This image will form on a screen or film.

REFLECTION occurs when a ray of light falling on a surface or an interface between two materials is turned back into the incident material.

REFRACTION occurs when a ray of light entering a material changes direction because of the difference in density between the incident and refracting materials.

RECTILINEAR PROPAGATION OF LIGHT is the law which says that light traveling through a homogeneous material travels in a straight line.

SAGITTAL DEPTH or SAG of a curve which has two endpoints is the least distance from the plane of the endpoints to the point of the curve farthest from this plane.

SECONDARY FOCAL POINT is the point on the optical axis toward which incident parallel paraxial rays will converge, or from which incident parallel paraxial rays appear to diverge, as a result of the lens or mirror.

SPECULAR REFLECTION is reflection from a surface that is smooth or polished.

SPHERICAL ABERRATION is the blurring of images that results from spherical lenses and mirrors having different focal lengths for rays of light that are not paraxial, or traveling near the axis. Peripheral rays come to a focus closer to the plane of the lens or mirror than paraxial rays do. This aberration is a problem only in optical systems with a large aperture. The iris of the eye, by limiting the size of the beam of light entering the eye, largely eliminates this aberration in ophthalmic applications. This aberration is a problem in instruments with wide aperture such as telescopes.

TORIC is a lens or surface which has different powers or curvatures in different meridians.

TRANSPARENCY is the attribute of a material which allows transmission of light to occur through the material without scattering the light.

TRANSVERSE WAVE MOTION occurs when the individual particles in the supporting material travel perpendicular to the direction of the propagation of the wave.

VERGENCE is a measurement of the relative direction of travel of two light rays. Vergence is the inverse of the distance the rays would have to travel in order to cross paths. See CONVERGENCE and DIVERGENCE.

VERTEX is the point where the axis of the lens or mirror intersects with the surface (either front or back) of the lens or mirror.

VIRTUAL IMAGE is an image which appears to be in a particular position, but is not, because the rays that form the image *appear* to be diverging from that position. This image will not form on a screen or film.

WAVELENGTH is the distance from a point on a wave to the corresponding point on the next wave.

Appendix 2
ANSI STANDARDS Z80.1 - 1999
Prescription Ophthalmic Lens Tolerance Recommendations

1. Tolerance for lens power:
   a. Definition: MERIDIONAL POWER: "The refractive or surface power of a lens measured in a specific meridian."
   b. Method of measurement: Focimeter, back or ocular surface of lens toward the lens stop. Power in the meridian of highest power must meet the following tolerance, based on the strongest power on the lens.
   Example: -6.00 -4.00 x090: the -10.00 power in the 180 meridian must fall within ±0.20D (2% of 10.00D)
   c. Tolerance: Individual single vision, aspheric design, traditional and progressive design multifocal designs:

Meridian of highest power	Tolerance on meridian of highest power
0.00 up to 6.50	±0.13
above 6.50	±2%

   Note: If the power has been compensated for wearing vertex distance, then the compensated power will be used to determine tolerances and the acceptable powers, and the documentation will indicate the compensated powers.
   Note: The test that was used in the 1995 standards for insuring that the sphere power and cylinder amount erred in the same direction has been replaced by the use of the highest meridian power for the meridional power tolerance instead of using the sphere power of the written prescription.

2. Tolerance for cylinder power:
   a. Definition: CYLINDER POWER: "The difference (plus or minus) between powers measured in the two principal meridians of a spherocylinder lens." A lens with spherical power is considered to have a cylinder of 0.00 D.
   b. Method of measurement: Focimeter, back surface of lens toward the lens stop. The difference between the two principal powers must meet the following tolerances, based on the amount of the cylinder power. **Example:** for -6.00 -4.00 x090, the difference between the 090 and 180 axis powers must be within ±0.15D.
   c. Individual single vision, aspheric design, traditional and progressive design multifocal designs:

Amount of cylinder	Tolerance on nominal value of the cylinder
0.00 up to 2.00	±0.13
above 2.00 up to 4.50	±0.15
above 4.50	±4%

3. Tolerance for cylinder axis:
   a. Definition: CYLINDER AXIS: "The principal meridian which contains only the spherical power component of a spherocylinder lens."

b. Method of measurement: Focimeter, back surface of lens toward the lens stop. **Example:** for -6.00 -4.00 x 090, the axis must be within 2 degrees of the 90th meridian.

c. Tolerances:

Nominal value of the cylinder power	Tolerance of the axis, in degrees
up to 0.37	±7
above 0.37 up to 0.75	±5
above 0.75 up to 1.50	±3
above 1.50	±2

4. Tolerance for addition power for multifocal and progressive addition lenses:
   a. Definition: ADDITION: "The difference in vertex power, referred to the surface containing the add, between the reading, or intermediate portion of a multifocal lens and its distance portion."
   b. Method of measurement: Focimeter, *surface of lens that contains the segment* toward the lens stop. Read either the sphere or cylinder power that gives target lines the closest to vertical for the distance, then the same lines for the near or intermediate portion. The difference between these two readings is the near addition. The distance reading should be taken as far above the DRP as the near reading is below the DRP, and outset the same amount as the near inset.

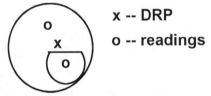

x -- DRP

o -- readings

   c. Tolerances:

Nominal value of addition power	Tolerance on the addition power
up to 4.00 D	±0.12
above 4.00 D	±0.18

   Note: If the addition power is compensated for wearing position or multifocal style, then the tolerance applies to the compensated value, and this compensated value must be documented. (Example: If the addition for a progressive lens is ordered 0.25 strong because of the progressive design, this compensation must be documented, and the tolerance applies to the new add power.).

5. Tolerance for prismatic power on a single lens:
   a. Definitions: PRISM REFERENCE POINT (PRP): "That point on a lens as specified by the manufacturer at which the prism value of the finished lens is to be measured."
   This differs from:
      The *fitting point*, which is the point on a lens (usually a progressive style lens) which is the reference point for positioning the lens; and from
      The *distance reference point* (DRP), which is the point on the lens where the sphere, cylinder and axis are to be measured. For an unmounted single vision lens this is generally the geometric center of the lens (unless the lens has prism ground for decentration). For multifocal lenses this point is referenced to the center of the

segment top and is determined by the segment drop and inset from frame geometrical center.

b. Method of measurement: For progressive addition lenses the PRP is the fitting point specified by the manufacturer, usually the dot below the fitting cross. For all other single vision and multifocal lenses, the PRP is the DRP. This point should be centered in the focimeter and the amount of prism present noted.

   i. VERTICAL IMBALANCE: The difference between the prism reference point height for the lenses must be no more than 1mm, or the induced prism resulting from different heights must be no more than $1/3^\Delta$.

   METHOD: Determine which of the two lenses has the greater absolute power on the 90th meridian. If powers are similar, determine which lens has the highest prescribed prism. Place this lens in the focimeter with the prism reference point centered and raise the lens table to the bottom of the glasses. Without changing the position of the lens table, move to the other lens and read the amount of vertical prism at that height. If there is more than $1/3^\Delta$, or, for prescribed prism, if the prism amount is more than $1/3^\Delta$ off, dot at this height, move this lens until the prism reference point is centered, and redot. If the dots are more than 1 mm apart the glasses do not meet specifications.
   See pages 84-85 in the text for a diagram of this method.

   ii. HORIZONTAL IMBALANCE: The difference between the prism reference points must be within 2.5mm of specification, or there may be up to $2/3^\Delta$ of unprescribed horizontal prism.

   METHOD: Dot prism reference points. If measurement is more than 2.5 mm from the specified amount, dot $1/3^\Delta$ of prism in each eye. (If measurement is too large, decenter lenses in for doting. If measurement is too small, decenter lenses out for doting.) Remeasure new dots. If new measurement is what was specified, or errs in the opposite direction from the original measurement, the mounted pair is acceptable.
   See pages 84-85 in the text for a diagram of this method.

c. Tolerances for mounted lenses:

Vertical power	Vertical
0.00 to 3.375 D	0.33^Δ in weaker lens
over 3.375 D	1 mm difference in heights

PROGRESSIVE ADDITION LENSES	
Horizontal power	Horizontal
0.00 to 3.375 D	0.67^Δ total on 180 meridian
over 3.375 D	1.0 mm difference from specified PRP

NON-PROGRESSIVE ADDITION LENSES	
Horizontal power	Horizontal
0.00 to 2.75 D	0.67^Δ total on 180 meridian
over 2.75 D	2.5 mm difference from specified distance PD

Note: Prism thinning is considered to be prescribed prism. For progressive addition lenses with power greater than 3.375 D, the *combined* vertical variation between the PRP may not exceed 1 mm..

6. Tolerance for BASE CURVE:
   a. Definition: ". . . marked or nominal tool surface power of the finished surface of a semi-finished spherical lens or the marked minimum tool surface power of the finished surface of a semi-finished toric lens."
   b. Method of measurement: For spherical surfaces, any method that is accurate to $\pm 0.25D$. Non aspheric and progressive design lenses might require calculations based on back surface curves, lens thickness, back vertex power, index of refraction (and the wavelength used to calculate the index of refraction).
   c. Tolerances: $\pm 0.75D$.

7. Tolerance for CENTER THICKNESS:
   a. Definition: "The thickness of a lens at the prism reference point." This tolerance is in effect when the thickness is specified by the prescriber or agreed to by the prescriber. There is **_no_** indication in the standards that this tolerance is an acceptable deviation from the safe thickness specified by the lens manufacturer for exemption of plastic lenses from impact resistance testing.
   b. Method of measurement: the thickness should be measured normal to the convex surface at the PRP.
   c. Tolerances: $\pm 0.3mm$

8. Tolerance for SEGMENT POSITION:
   a. Definition of segment: "A specified area of a multifocal lens having a different refractive power from the distance portion."
   b. Method of measurement: Based on the boxing system of measurement.
   c. Tolerances:
      i. Vertical placement:
         - The segment top for a non-progressive addition lens, or the fitting cross of a progressive addition lens, must be within $\pm 1mm$ of specification.
         - The difference between the two segment heights in a mounted pair may not exceed 1mm unless specified otherwise.
      ii. Horizontal placement:
         - For a mounted pair, the centers of the tops of the segments must be within $\pm 2.5mm$ of the near interpupillary distance specification. There is no 0.67^Δ exemption for the placement of the multifocal segment in low power non-progressive addition lenses.
         - The segments will appear symmetrical unless requested otherwise.
         - For progressive addition lenses, the fitting cross and the distance interpupillary distance will be used, and each individual lens will vary by on more than 1 mm from the monocular specification.

9. Requirements for claiming UV protection:
   a. Definitions: UV_B is between 290 and 315nm. UV_A is between 315 and 380nm.
   b. Method of measurement: Mathematical. Practical method not specified.
   c. Specifications: "Manufacturers of lenses who claim specific ultraviolet attenuating properties shall state the average percent transmittance between 290 and 315nm (UV_B) and between 315 and 380 nm (UV_A)."

Optical Formulas Tutorial

10. Warpage and waves:
   a. Definitions: A wave would result in a straight line appearing curved when viewed through the lens. Warpage is a lens defect that is the result of improper processing or mounting.
   b. Method of measurement: Looking at a grid of straight lines through the lens held at either arm's length or with the inspector's eye at 12 inches (for weak power lenses) or at the focal length of the lens will aid the inspector in noticing areas that should be checked in the focimeter. Warpage can be checked with a lens clock or sagitta gauge.
   c. Tolerances:
   - Noticeable focimeter target distortion or blur is not acceptable within 15mm radius of the DRP in any direction.
   - If the segment is more than 30mm then there should be no distortion or blur within 15mm of the center of the top of the segment. For segments smaller than 30mm there may be no distortion or blur over the whole area of the segment.
   - Warpage of the base curve that is the result of finished processing will not exceed 1D.
   - Distortion or blur is acceptable outside of the optical area of both lenticular lenses and progressive power lenses.
   - These requirements are waived within 6mm of the edge of the lens.

11. IMPACT RESISTANCE: "All lenses must conform to the impact resistance requirements. . . Laminated, plastic and raised-ledge multifocal lenses may be certified by the manufacturer as conforming to the initial design testing or statistically significant sampling. . . All monolithic (not laminated) glass lenses shall be treated to be resistant to impact."
   METHOD: 5/8 in (15.9mm) diameter steel ball weighing not less than 0.56oz (16 grams) dropped from no less than 50 inches (127cm). Lens should be centered, but multifocal lenses may be decentered so that the ball will not impact the segment. Lenses should not be clamped. The lens may be covered by or placed in a bag of polyethylene, no heavier than 0.076mm or 0.003in thick. This protection should be in contact with the lens surface during the test.
   EXEMPTIONS: The following are exempted from the drop-ball technique of testing:
   prism segment multifocals
   slab-off prisms
   lenticular cataracts
   iseikonics
   depressed segment one-piece multifocals
   biconcaves, myodiscs and minus lenticulars
   custom laminates and cemented assemblies

Note: All quotes, tables, definitions, methodology and tolerances were taken from American National Standard Z80.1-1999, copyright © 2000 by Optical Laboratories Association, and with the permission of the Optical Laboratories Association. The standards are published by the Optical Laboratories Association, P.O. Box 2000, Merrifield, VA, 22116-2000. Data is accurate as of publication.

Appendix 3
OPTICAL SYMBOLS AND FORMULAS

The following symbols are used in the formulas in this appendix. Any other symbol used in a formula will be defined in the formula. Page references are to the beginning of the discussion of the formula.

a = apical angle.
d = distance in mm or m.
D = diopters.
δ = angle of deviation.
f = focal length in meters.
i = angle of incidence.
I = intensity of light.
λ = wavelength of a light wave in nm.

M = magnification in decimal form.
n = refractive index.
p = object distance.
P = prism diopters.
q = image distance.
r = angle of refraction or angle of reflection.
r = radius of curvature in meters.
t = thickness in meters.

ABBE VALUE page 26.

$$v = \frac{(n_{yellow} - 1)}{(n_{blue} - n_{red})}$$

$v = nu$ value or constringence,

ANTI-REFLECTIVE COATINGS page 140, 141.

$$(n_{coating})^2 = n_{lens}$$ Ideal coating material; not practical.

$$\text{coating thickness} = {}^{m}/_{\lambda},$$ where λ is the wavelength of a particular wave; m = 1,3,5,7...; m=1 is ideal.

BACK VERTEX POWER page 151.

$$D_{back} = D_2 + \frac{D_1}{1 - ({}^{t}/_{n})D_1}$$ (exact formula, t is thickness in meters.)

$$D_{back} \approx D_1 + D_2 + ({}^{t}/_{n})(D_1)^2$$ (approximation; t is thickness in meters.)

See also EQUIVALENT POWER, FRONT VERTEX POWER, OPTICAL CENTER.

BASE CURVE or VOGEL'S RULE page 114.
plus lens: front base curve = spherical equivalent + 6.00
minus lens: front base curve = 1/2 spherical equivalent + 6.00

BREWSTER'S ANGLE page 147.
$$\tan i = n_i/n_r$$

Optical Formulas Tutorial

CARDINAL POINTS: see EQUIVALENT POWER,
FRONT and BACK VERTEX POWER,
NODAL POINTS, PRINCIPAL PLANE.

CIRCLE OF LEAST CONFUSION: see SPHERICAL EQUIVALENT.

COMPENSATED POWER page 68.

$$D_{new} = \frac{D_{Rx}}{(1 - dD_{Rx})}$$

(where d is the change in vertex distance; it is negative if lens is moved away from eye, positive if lens is moved toward the eye.)

See also EFFECTIVE POWER.

CRITICAL ANGLE page 24.

$$\sin i = n_r/n_i$$

See also SNELL's LAW.

CROSSED CYLINDERS: see THOMPSON'S FORMULA.

DIFFRACTION page 149

$$\lambda = \frac{dy}{l}$$

d = distance between slits in diffraction grating, meters
y = distance between first two areas of constructive interference
l = distance from diffraction grating to screen, meters

DIOPTERS OF PRISM: see PRISM.

DISPERSIVE POWER: inverse of ABBE NUMBER.

EFFECTIVE POWER page 65.

$$D_{effective} = \frac{D_{Rx}}{(1 + dD_{Rx})}$$

(where d is the change in vertex distance; it is negative if lens is moved away from eye, positive if lens is moved toward the eye.)

See also COMPENSATED POWER.

EQUIVALENT POWER page 170.

$$D_{eq} = D_1 + D_2 + (^t/_n)D_1D_2 \quad \text{(t is thickness in meters.)}$$

See also BACK and FRONT VERTEX POWER.

FOCAL LENGTH FORMULA page 29.

$$D = \frac{n_i}{f} \qquad f = \frac{n_i}{D} \qquad f \approx \frac{40(n_i)}{D} \text{ for f in inches.}$$

In general, $n_i = 1$.

FRESNEL'S EQUATION FOR REFLECTION page 137.

$$I_r = \frac{(n-1)^2}{(n+1)^2}$$

I_r = amount of light reflected from one surface, in decimal form.

FRONT VERTEX POWER page 152.

$$D_{front} = D_1 + \frac{D_2}{1 - (^t/_n)D_2}$$

(exact formula, t is thickness in meters.)

$$D_{front} \approx D_1 + D_2 + (^t/_n)(D_2)^2$$

(approximation; t is thickness in meters.)

See also EQUIVALENT POWER, OPTICAL CENTER, BACK VERTEX POWER.

ILLUMINATION page 16.

$$E = ^I/_{d^2}$$

E = illumination on object in lux (or foot candles)

I = light emitted or reflected from source

d = distance of object from source in meters (or feet)

IMAGE PLACEMENT, LENS OR SPHERICAL MIRROR page 158.

$$^1/_f = ^1/_p + ^1/_q$$

p = object distance, q = image distance

See text for sign conventions.

See also MAGNIFICATION. See page 183 for most general form.

INDEX OF REFRACTION page 22.

$$n = \frac{\text{speed of light in a vacuum}}{\text{speed of light in material}}$$

Also called Mu, μ.

LAMBERT'S EQUATION for lens transmission page 144.

$$I_2 = I_1 T^q$$

I_2 = transmission through an absorptive glass lens,

I_1 = percent of light entering the absorptive glass lens,

T = transmission per 2mm of lens material

q = thickness of lens in mm/2.

LENSMAKER'S EQUATION page 36.

$$D = +/- \frac{n-1}{r_1} +/- \frac{n-1}{r_2}$$

(+ for convex surfaces, – for concave surfaces)

General case, where lens is surrounded by air.

See also SURFACE POWER FORMULA.

MAGNIFICATION page 158.
$$M = -\frac{p}{q} = \frac{I}{O} \text{ (lenses \& mirror linear magnification.)}$$
See also IMAGE PLACEMENT, SPECTACLE MAGNIFICATION.

MALUS' LAW page 148.
$$I_2 = I_1 \cos^2\theta$$
θ is the difference in orientation of two polarizing filters to each other.

MARTIN'S FORMULA FOR PANTOSCOPIC TILT page 127.
$$D_{sph} = D(1 + \frac{\sin^2\alpha}{2n})$$
α = degrees of tilt,
D = sphere power on the 180 meridian
D_{sph} = induced sphere,
$$D_{cyl} = D_{sph} \tan^2\alpha$$
D_{cyl} = induced cylinder on the 180.

To eliminate unwanted induced power and cylinder, lower OC 1mm for every 2° pantoscopic tilt.

MINIMUM BLANK SIZE page 112.
minimum blank size = ED + total decentration + 2
= ED + 2×(one-lens decentration) + 2

MIRRORS: see IMAGE PLACEMENT and MAGNIFICATION.

n: see INDEX OF REFRACTION.

NODAL POINTS page 181.
$$HN = H_2f_2 - f_1H_1$$
HN is distance from principal point to corresponding nodal point. See text.
See also PRINCIPAL PLANE, EQUIVALENT POWER, FRONT and BACK VERTEX POWER.

NOMINAL POWER FORMULA page 33.
$$D_n = D_1 + D_2 \quad (D_1 \text{ and } D_2 \text{ are front and back surface powers})$$

OBLIQUE MERIDIAN page 62.
$$D_T = D_{sph} + D_{cyl}\sin^2\alpha$$
α = difference between axis of Rx and oblique meridian wanted.

OBLIQUELY CROSSED CYLINDERS: see THOMPSON'S FORMULA.

OPTICAL CENTER, THICK LENSES page 170.
$$V_1O = (r_1t)/(r_1 - r_2)$$
V_1O is distance from front vertex to optical center.

PANTOSCOPIC TILT: see MARTIN'S FORMULA.

POLARIZING FILTERS: see MALUS' LAW.

PRENTICE'S RULE page 79.

$$P = \frac{dD}{10}$$ (where d is in mm.)

PRINCIPAL PLANE page 170.

$V_1H_1 = f - f_1$ f derived from D_{eq}, f_1 derived from D_F, f_2 from D_B

$V_2H_2 = f_2 - f$ V_1H_1 distance, front vertex to first principal plane.

V_2H_2 distance, back vertex to second principal plane.

PRISM page 73, 75 ,76.

$$\delta = a(n-1)$$ δ is angle of deviation, a is apical angle.

$$P = \frac{\text{displacement of image in cm}}{\text{distance from prism in meters}}$$

$$P = 100 \tan \delta = 100 \tan [a(n-1)]$$

See also PRENTICE'S RULE, PRISM THICKNESS, RESULTANT PRISM, RESOLVING PRISM.

PRISM THICKNESS page 123.

$$t = \frac{dP}{100(n-1)} \qquad P = \frac{t(100[n-1])}{d}$$

t = base to apex difference, in mm.

d = lens diameter, mm.

(Note: for a 50mm blank, if n = 1.50, then there is 1mm thickness per 1^Δ prism.)
See also PRISM.

RECOMPUTED POWER: see EFFECTIVE POWER and COMPENSATED POWER.

REFLECTION, LAW OF page 19.

angle of incidence = angle of reflection
See also FRESNEL'S EQUATION FOR REFLECTION.

REFRACTION, LAW OF: see SNELL'S LAW.

RESOLVING PRISM page 103.

V = (P)(sin a)   a = angle of orientation of prism.
H = (P)(cos a)   Ignore sign of sin a and cos a.
See also RESULTANT PRISM.

RESULTANT PRISM page 99.

$$P^2 = V^2 + H^2$$

$$\tan a = \frac{V}{H}$$

180–a	a
180+a	360–a

See also RESOLVING PRISM.

Optical Formulas Tutorial

SAG page 119, 122.

$$\text{sag} = r - \sqrt{r^2 - \left(\frac{d}{2}\right)^2}$$

(where d is eyesize, minimum blank size, or diameter of the lens.)
All units in mm, cm, or m. (All the same.)

Approximation formula:

$$\text{sag} \approx \frac{(d/2)^2 D}{2000(n-1)}$$

(where d is eyesize, minimum blank size, or diameter of the lens, in mm.)

See also THICKNESS FORMULA.

SNELL'S LAW page 23, 21.

$$n_i \sin i = n_r \sin r$$

$$i = r + \delta$$

See also CRITICAL ANGLE.

SPECTACLE MAGNIFICATION page 130.

$$\text{SM} = \frac{1}{1 - (^t/_n)D_1} \times \frac{1}{1 - hD}$$

h = vertex distance + .003, in meters

change in magnification, approximations:

$$\Delta\%\text{SM} = \Delta D_1 t/15$$

$$\Delta\%\text{SM} = D_1 \Delta t/15$$

$$\Delta\%\text{SM} = \Delta hD/10$$

(All measurements in mm. Gives approximate change in percent magnification, based on single changes. See text for explanations. Δ means **"change in."**)

SPHERICAL EQUIVALENT page 54.

$$D_{\text{sph. eq.}} = D_{\text{sphere}} + \frac{D_{\text{cyl}}}{2}$$

SURFACE POWER FORMULA page 35, 168.

$$D = \frac{n_r - n_i}{r}$$

(r + if center of curvature is to the right of the surface, r − if center of curvature is to the left of the surface.)

See also **LENSMAKER'S EQUATION.**

THICKNESS FORMULA page 122.

plus lens: center thickness = edge thickness + sag$_{\text{lens}}$
minus lens: edge thickness = center thickness + sag$_{\text{lens}}$

See also SAG, PRISM THICKNESS.

THICK LENS FORMULA: see BACK & FRONT VERTEX POWER, EQUIVALENT POWER, NODAL POINTS, OPTICAL CENTER, PRINCIPAL PLANES.

THIN LENS: see IMAGE PLACEMENT and MAGNIFICATION.

THOMPSON'S FORMULA for OBLIQUELY CROSSED CYLINDERS page 135.

$$C^2 = C_1^2 + C_2^2 + 2C_1C_2\cos2\gamma$$

$$S = S_1 + S_2 + \frac{C_1 + C_2 - C}{2}$$

$$\tan 2\theta = \frac{C_2\sin2\gamma}{C_1 + C_2\cos2\gamma}$$

Convert both Rx's to plus cylinder, label the Rx with the lower axis $S_1\ C_1\ \text{axis}_1$ and the Rx with the higher axis $S_2\ C_2\ \text{axis}_2$.

γ is $\text{axis}_2 - \text{axis}_1$.

θ is added to axis_1.

See pages 135-137 for more explanation.

TILT: see MARTIN'S FORMULA.

TRUE POWER FORMULA page 117.

$$\frac{D_{(marked)}}{D_{(true)}} = \frac{0.530}{n-1}$$

or

$$D_{(true)} = \frac{n-1}{0.530}\ D_{(marked)}$$

or

$$D_{(marked)} = \frac{0.530}{n-1}\ D_{(true)}$$

VOGEL'S RULE page 114.

plus lens: front base curve = spherical equivalent + 6.00

minus lens: front base curve = 1/2 spherical equivalent + 6.00

WAVE FORMULA page 13.

$v = f\lambda$ v = velocity of light in the medium, in meters/second.

f = frequency of the wave in Hz (waves/second).

λ = wavelength of the wave in the medium, in meters/wave.

Appendix 4
TRIGONOMETRIC TABLES

angle	sine (sin)	cosine (cos)	tangent (tan)	angle	sine (sin)	cosine (cos)	tangent (tan)
0	0.00000	1.00000	0.00000				
1	0.01745	0.99985	0.01746	46	0.71934	0.69466	1.03553
2	0.03490	0.99939	0.03492	47	0.73135	0.68200	1.07237
3	0.05234	0.99863	0.05241	48	0.74315	0.66913	1.11061
4	0.06976	0.99756	0.06993	49	0.75471	0.65606	1.15037
5	0.08716	0.99619	0.08749	50	0.76604	0.64279	1.19175
6	0.10453	0.99452	0.10510	51	0.77715	0.62932	1.23490
7	0.12187	0.99255	0.12278	52	0.78801	0.61566	1.27994
8	0.13917	0.99027	0.14054	53	0.79864	0.60181	1.32705
9	0.15643	0.98769	0.15838	54	0.80902	0.58778	1.37638
10	0.17365	0.98481	0.17633	55	0.81915	0.57358	1.42815
11	0.19081	0.98163	0.19438	56	0.82904	0.55919	1.48256
12	0.20791	0.97815	0.21256	57	0.83867	0.54464	1.53987
13	0.22495	0.97437	0.23087	58	0.84805	0.52992	1.60034
14	0.24192	0.97030	0.24933	59	0.85717	0.51504	1.66428
15	0.25882	0.96593	0.26795	60	0.86603	0.50000	1.73205
16	0.27564	0.96126	0.28675	61	0.87462	0.48481	1.80405
17	0.29237	0.95630	0.30573	62	0.88295	0.46947	1.88073
18	0.30902	0.95106	0.32492	63	0.89101	0.45399	1.96261
19	0.32557	0.94552	0.34433	64	0.89879	0.43837	2.05031
20	0.34202	0.93969	0.36397	65	0.90631	0.42262	2.14451
21	0.35837	0.93358	0.38386	66	0.91355	0.40674	2.24604
22	0.37461	0.92718	0.40403	67	0.92051	0.39073	2.35586
23	0.39073	0.92050	0.42448	68	0.92718	0.37461	2.47509
24	0.40674	0.91355	0.44523	69	0.93358	0.35837	2.60509
25	0.42262	0.90631	0.46631	70	0.93969	0.34202	2.747481
26	0.43837	0.89879	0.48773	71	0.94552	0.32557	2.90422
27	0.45399	0.89101	0.50953	72	0.95106	0.30902	3.07769
28	0.46947	0.88295	0.53171	73	0.95630	0.29237	3.27086
29	0.48481	0.87462	0.55431	74	0.96126	0.27564	3.48742
30	0.50000	0.86603	0.57735	75	0.96593	0.25882	3.73206
31	0.51504	0.85717	0.60086	76	0.97030	0.24192	4.01079
32	0.52992	0.84805	0.62487	77	0.97437	0.22495	4.33149
33	0.54464	0.83867	0.64941	78	0.97815	0.20791	4.70464
34	0.55919	0.82904	0.67451	79	0.98163	0.19081	5.14457
35	0.57358	0.81915	0.70021	80	0.98481	0.17365	5.67130
36	0.58779	0.80902	0.72654	81	0.98769	0.15643	6.31378
37	0.60182	0.79864	0.75355	82	0.99027	0.13917	7.11540
38	0.61566	0.78801	0.78129	83	0.99255	0.12187	8.14439
39	0.62932	0.77715	0.80978	84	0.99452	0.10453	9.51442
40	0.64279	0.76604	0.83910	85	0.99619	0.08716	11.43014
41	0.65606	0.75471	0.86929	86	0.99756	0.06976	14.30080
42	0.66913	0.74314	0.90040	87	0.99863	0.05234	19.08137
43	0.68200	0.73135	0.93252	88	0.99939	0.03490	28.63679
44	0.69466	0.71934	0.96569	89	0.99985	0.01745	57.29215
45	0.70711	0.70711	1.00000	90	1.00000	0.00000	not defined

angle	sine (sin)	cosine (cos)	tangent (tan)	angle	sine (sin)	cosine (cos)	tangent (tan)
91	0.99985	-0.01745	-57.28996	136	0.69466	-0.71934	-0.96569
92	0.99939	-0.03490	-28.63625	137	0.68200	-0.73135	-0.93252
93	0.99863	-0.05234	-19.08114	138	0.66913	-0.74314	-0.90040
94	0.99756	-0.06976	-14.30067	139	0.65606	-0.75471	-0.86929
95	0.99619	-0.08716	-11.43005	140	0.64279	-0.76604	-0.83910
96	0.99452	-0.10453	-9.51436	141	0.62932	-0.77715	-0.80978
97	0.99255	-0.12187	-8.14435	142	0.61566	-0.78801	-0.78129
98	0.99027	-0.13917	-7.11537	143	0.60182	-0.79864	-0.75355
99	0.98769	-0.15643	-6.31375	144	0.58779	-0.80902	-0.72654
100	0.98481	-0.17365	-5.67128	145	0.57358	-0.81915	-0.70021
101	0.98163	-0.19081	-5.14455	146	0.55919	-0.82904	-0.67451
102	0.97815	-0.20791	-4.70463	147	0.54464	-0.83867	-0.64941
103	0.97437	-0.22495	-4.33148	148	0.52992	-0.84805	-0.62487
104	0.97030	-0.24192	-4.01078	149	0.51504	-0.85717	-0.60086
105	0.96593	-0.25882	-3.73205	150	0.50000	-0.86603	-0.57735
106	0.96126	-0.27564	-3.48741	151	0.48481	-0.87462	-0.55431
107	0.95630	-0.29237	-3.27085	152	0.46947	-0.88295	-0.53171
108	0.95106	-0.30902	-3.07768	153	0.45399	-0.89101	-0.50953
109	0.94552	-0.32557	-2.90421	154	0.43837	-0.89879	-0.48773
110	0.93969	-0.34202	-2.74748	155	0.42262	-0.90631	-0.46631
111	0.93358	-0.35837	-2.60509	156	0.40674	-0.91355	-0.44523
112	0.92718	-0.37461	-2.47509	157	0.39073	-0.92050	-0.42447
113	0.92050	-0.39073	-2.35585	158	0.37461	-0.92718	-0.40403
114	0.91355	-0.40674	-2.24604	159	0.35837	-0.93358	-0.38386
115	0.90631	-0.42262	-2.14451	160	0.34202	-0.93969	-0.36397
116	0.89879	-0.43837	-2.05030	161	0.32557	-0.94552	-0.34433
117	0.89101	-0.45399	-1.96261	162	0.30902	-0.95106	-0.32492
118	0.88295	-0.46947	-1.88073	163	0.29237	-0.95630	-0.30573
119	0.87462	-0.48481	-1.80405	164	0.27564	-0.96126	-0.28675
120	0.86603	-0.50000	-1.73205	165	0.25882	-0.96593	-0.26795
121	0.85717	-0.51504	-1.66428	166	0.24192	-0.97030	-0.24933
122	0.84805	-0.52992	-1.60033	167	0.22495	-0.97437	-0.23087
123	0.83867	-0.54464	-1.53986	168	0.20791	-0.97815	-0.21256
124	0.82904	-0.55919	-1.48256	169	0.19081	-0.98163	-0.19438
125	0.81915	-0.57358	-1.42815	170	0.17365	-0.98481	-0.17633
126	0.80902	-0.58779	-1.37638	171	0.15643	-0.98769	-0.15838
127	0.79864	-0.60182	-1.32704	172	0.13917	-0.99027	-0.14054
128	0.78801	-0.61566	-1.27994	173	0.12187	-0.99255	-0.12278
129	0.77715	-0.62932	-1.23490	174	0.10453	-0.99452	-0.10510
130	0.76604	-0.64279	-1.19175	175	0.08716	-0.99619	-0.08749
131	0.75471	-0.65606	-1.15037	176	0.06976	-0.99756	-0.06993
132	0.74314	-0.66913	-1.11061	177	0.05234	-0.99863	-0.05241
133	0.73135	-0.68200	-1.07237	178	0.03490	-0.99939	-0.03492
134	0.71934	-0.69466	-1.03553	179	0.01745	-0.99985	-0.01746
135	0.70711	-0.70711	-1.00000	180	0.00000	-1.00000	0.00000

Appendix 5
REFERENCES

American Optical 4 book set of programmed instruction. *Basic Optical Concepts; Normal and Abnormal Vision; The Human Eye; Lenses, Prisms and Mirrors.* Southbridge, Mass.: AO, 1986.

ANSI Standards, Z80.1-1995, 11 West 42nd Street, New York, NY 10036.

Brooks, *Essentials for Ophthalmic Lens Work.* Professional Press, 1983.

Brooks, *Understanding Lens Surfacing.* Boston: Butterworth-Heinemann, 1992.

Brooks and Borish, *System for Ophthalmic Dispensing, 2nd ed.* Boston: Butterworth-Heinemann, 1995.

Coletta, *College Physics.* St. Louis: Mosby, 1995.

Crummett and Western, *University Physics, Models and Applications.* Dubuque, Iowa: W.C. Brown, 1994.

Epting and Morgret, Jr. *Ophthalmic Mechanics and Dispensing.* Radnor, Pa.: Chilton Book Co, 1964.

Ervin, ed. *The Masters Review.* N.A.O.

Fannin and Grosvenor, *Clinical Optics, 2nd ed.* Boston: Butterworth-Heinemann, 1996.

Farrell, *The Glossary of Optical Terminology.* New York: Professional Press, 1986.

Freemen, *Optics.* 10th ed. London: Butterworths, 1990.

Jalie, *The Principles of Ophthalmic Lenses.* London: Association of Dispensing Opticians, 1980.

Janney and Tunnacliffe, *Worked Problems in Ophthalmic Lenses.* London: Eastern Press Ltd., 1979.

Jenkins and White, *Fundamentals of Optics.* New York: McGraw-Hill, 1957.

Keeney, Hagman, and Fratello, *Dictionary of Ophthalmic Optics.* N.A.O., 1995.

Loshin, *The Geometrical Optics Workbook.* Boston: Butterworth-Heinemann, 1991.

Meyer-Aremdt, *Introduction to Classical and Modern Optics.* Englewood Cliffs, NJ: Prentice-Hall, 1995.

N.A.O., *Career Progression Program.* Bowie, Maryland: National Academy of Opticianry.

Pedrotti and Pedrotti, *Introduction to Optics.* Englewood Cliffs, NJ: Prentice-Hall, 1993.

Rubin, *Optics for Clinicians.* 2nd ed. Gainesville, Fl: TRIAD Scientific, 1977.

Saude, *Ocular Anatomy and Physiology.* Boston: Blackwell Scientific, 1993.

Stein, Slatt, and Stein, *Fitting Guide for Rigid and Soft Contact Lenses.* St. Louis: Mosby, 1990.

Appendix 6
ANSWERS TO EXERCISES

Section I

page 1 Addition	page 2 Subtraction	page 2-3 Multiplication	page 3 Division
1. +2.00	1. 0	1. +1.00	1. +1.00
2. −2.00	2. 0	2. +1.00	2. +1.00
3. +4.50	3. +1.50	3. +4.50	3. +2.00
4. +1.50	4. +4.50	4. −4.50	4. −2.00
5. −6.50	5. −2.50	5. +9.00	5. +2.25
6. −2.50	6. −6.50	6. −9.00	6. −2.25
7. +1.50	7. +13.50	7. −45.00	7. −1.25
8. +4.87	8. −11.37	8. −26.39	8. −0.40
9. −14.50	9. −5.50	9. +45.00	9. +2.22
10. +8.00	10. +5.50	10. +8.4375	10. +5.40

page 4	page 5	page 6
1. 132.57	1. 5000mm	1. 6.10in
2. 0.46	2. 200cm	2. 0.51ft
3. 1.56	3. 500mm	3. 1.83m
4. 6	4. 0.2cm	4. 6.1m
5. 4	5. 0.00245m	5. 4.72in
6. 9	6. 45mm	6. 40.64cm
7. −6.62	7. 0.045m	7. 0.76m
8. +0.25	8. 0.0805m	8. 3.28ft
9. −3.25		

page 8

1. 0.58779
2. 0.01745
3. 0.01746
4. 0
5. −0.80902
6. −28.63625
7. 36 degrees
8. 54 degrees
9. 20 degrees
10. −20 from calculator, 160 from tables.
11. 99 degrees
12. 30 degrees. The tables also give 150 degrees.
13. 0.50

Section II

page 14	page 17	page 21	page 23
1. 5.10×10^{14}	1. a. 63 lux	1. r = 15°	1. n = 1.58
2. 371nm	b. 40 lux	2. i = 15°	2. n = 1.71
3. 442nm	2. 3,333,333 lux	3. $\delta = -18°$	3. 122,000 mps
4. 360nm; UV-A	1,875,000 lux	(leaving denser mat'l)	
		4. r = 29°	

page 24	page 25	page 27
1. 61°	1. 36°	1. V = 29
2. 18°	2. a. 23°, b. 39°,	*n = 1.72
3. 28°	c. 59°, d. reflects, e. reflects	
	3. 33°	

Section III

page 30-31

1. +20.00D
2. +10 in. (actual 9.8in.)
3. −0.2m or −20cm
4. +2.50D
5. +10.00D
6. +5.00D

page 34-35

1. +6.00D / flat / bi-convex
    or equi-convex
2. −4.50D / bent / meniscus
3. −10.00D / flat / bi-concave

4. +4.75D
5. +7.62D
6. −5.25D
7. +5.00D
8. −6.00D

page 37

1. −5.62D
2. −1.87D (periscopic)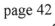
3. +3.50D in n=1.60;   +2.87D in CR39

page 42

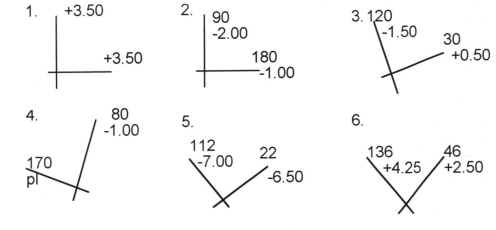

page 45 - 47

1a. −0.50 −0.50 x135
 b. +3.00 −4.50 x080
 c. −0.50 −1.00 x090
 d. +3.50 −1.00 x110
 e. +2.12 −2.00 x175
 f. +12.00DS

2a. −1.00 +0.50 x045
 b. −1.50 +4.50 x170
 c. −1.50 +1.00 x180
 d. +2.50 +1.00 x020
3a. +2.50 x020 ⚬ −1.00 x110 (any order)
 b. +1.00 x030 ⚬ −1.00 x120 (any order)

* The values are taken from Meyer-Arendt, *Introduction to Classical and Modern Optics,* page 19.

     1a. +1.00 −1.50 x120   2a. −1.00 +3.00 x150

      b. +4.00 −3.00 x045   b. −1.75 +0.75 x050

      c. −0.87 −1.50 x160   c. −3.37 +1.75 x155

page 49 (Cross cylinders may be in any order.)

     1a. −1.00 x180 ☎ +1.00 x090   2a. +2.00 −3.00 x110

      b. +2.50 x040 ☎ −1.12 x130   b. +3.25 −2.25 x170

      c. +1.00 x006 ☎ −0.50 x096   c. +10.50 −1.00 x103

page 50-51

     1. +4.00 −2.00 x180   or   +2.00 +2.00 x090

     2. −4.00 −2.00 x180   or   −6.00 +2.00 x090

     3. +1.00 −3.50 x090   or   −2.50 +3.50 x180

     4. +1.50 −0.50 x135   or   +1.00 + 0.50 x045

page 52 (corrections underlined.)

     1. <u>+8.50</u> −1.00 x<u>015</u>   6. <u>pl</u> +0.62 x<u>010</u>   11. −<u>7.50D</u> or −7.50DS

     2. <u>+/−</u>3.50 +1.50 x135   7. correct   12. <u>+0.62 −0.62</u> x<u>010</u>

        (call the prescriber)   8. −3.00 <u>+/−</u>0.75 x015   13. <u>−3.12</u> +<u>3.12</u> x067

     3. <u>−0.37</u> −1.50 x<u>008</u>   (call the prescriber)   14. <u>−1.12D</u> or −1.12DS

     4. correct   9. correct   15. +0.50 −0.50 x<u>030</u>

     5. <u>+3.75D</u> or +3.75DS   10. correct   16. correct

page 54-55

     1. −1.25D

     2. −1.00D

     3. +0.50D

     4. −0.62D

     5. +2.00D

     6. +0.25D

     7. +2.50D

     8. −1.62D

     9. −1.37D

     10. −2.50D

page 58

     1. MA

     2. M

     3. CMA

     4. SHA

     5. H

     6. CHA

     7. MA

     8. SMA

page 59

     1. CMA

     2. SMA

     3. MA

     4. SMA

     5. CHA

     6. MA

     7. CHA

     8. CMA

     9. CHA

     10. SHA

page 61

     1. WR

     2. O

     3. WR

     4. AR

     5. WR

     6. O

     7. WR

     8. WR

     9. O

     10. AR

page 63

     1. −0.50D

     2. −6.00D

     3. +2.25D

     4. +1.00DC

        (power −1.50D)

     5. +4.71D

     6. −9.48D

page 67

1. OD −5.26D (effective)   2. OD +5.15 +2.16 x090 (effective)
   OS −6.95D (effective)   OS +6.22 +2.74 x145 (effective)

page 70

1. OD −4.75D (rounded)   2. OD +4.87 +1.87 x090 (rounded)
   OS −6.00 (rounded; −6.12 not avail.) OS +5.75 +2.37 x145 (rounded)
3a. −6.38 −1.91 x090 (effective)   3b. −6.62 −2.12 x090 (rounded)
     −8.05 −0.24 x090 (effective)   −8.50 −0.25 x090 (rounded)
3c. −6.00 −1.75 x090   3d. −6.75 −2.25 x090 (rounded)
     −7.75DS (if available)   −8.75 −0.25 x090 (rounded)

Section IV

page 73   page 76

1. $\delta = 11.9°$ 1. $1^{\triangle}$ base to the right
2. $a = 36.1°$ 2. 8cm (movement is down)
3. $n = 1.60$ 3. 1.5m, base up

page 77   page 81

1. 2.0°   1. $0.8^{\triangle}$, BU
2. 4.0°   2. 0
3. $n = 1.60$ 3. $1.4^{\triangle}$BO
               4. $2.8^{\triangle}$BU

page 84   page 86

1. OD $0.7^{\triangle}$ BI   2. total $0.1^{\triangle}$ BI   1. OD $1.5^{\triangle}$BU OS $1.5^{\triangle}$BD
    OS $0.4^{\triangle}$ BO   3. total $2.8^{\triangle}$ BI   2. OD $2^{\triangle}$BI OS $2^{\triangle}$BI
      total prism   4. $1.3^{\triangle}$ BU OD or BD OS   3. OD $1.5^{\triangle}$BO OS $1.5^{\triangle}$BO
      $0.3^{\triangle}$ BI OD   5. $0.6^{\triangle}$BI; yes;$1.5^{\triangle}$BI;no   4. OD $2.5^{\triangle}$BU OS $2.5^{\triangle}$BD

page 88-89   page 94

1. $1.3^{\triangle}$BD OU   1. Difference needed 6mm
2. $0^{\triangle}$ OU   use FT OD and rnd 22 OS
3. $2.5^{\triangle}$BD OD $3.3^{\triangle}$BD OS   or Exec/PAL OD and FT OS

page 95

1. total $2.6^{\triangle}$ BD OD, order $2.6^{\triangle}$ slab-off OD or $2.6^{\triangle}$ reverse slab-off OS.
2. total $3.2^{\triangle}$ BU OD, order $3.2^{\triangle}$ slab-off OS or $3.2^{\triangle}$ reverse slab-off OD.
3. total $2.8^{\triangle}$ BD OS, order $2.8^{\triangle}$ slab-off OS or $2.8^{\triangle}$ reverse slab-off OD.

page 101   b. OD   e. OS

page 102-103

1. $3.2^{\triangle}$ BU&I @ 045 or $3.2^{\triangle}$ @ 045
2. $2.2^{\triangle}$ BU&I @ 117 or $2.2^{\triangle}$ @ 117

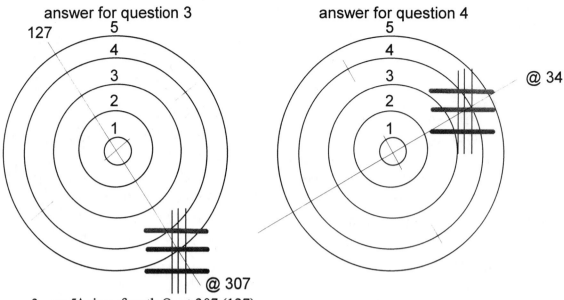

answer for question 3

answer for question 4

127

@ 34

@ 307

3. on 5$^\Delta$ ring, fourth Q, at 307 (127)
4. 3.6$^\Delta$ @034; therefore it would be drawn a little more than
    1/2 way between the 3 and 4 rings, 1st quadrant, @34.

page 104

1. 2.2$^\Delta$ BD & 0.6$^\Delta$ BO
2. 3$^\Delta$ BD & 3$^\Delta$ BI
3. 2.3$^\Delta$ BU&O @50 becomes 1.8$^\Delta$ BU & 1.5$^\Delta$ BO

Section V

page 111		frame 1	frame 2	frame 3
a.	A	48	53	61/60
	B	31	42	43
	DBL	13	13	5
	FPD	61	66	66
	ED	51	58	61
	P	17	11	18/17
b.	D	48	50	61/60
	DBL	13	18	5
c.	Seg height	19	24/23	18.5
	below/above	above3.5	above3&2	below3
d.		0	2.5	2.5
e.		1.5in&1.5out	4in&1in	4in&1in

page 113	page 115	page 116
1. 67mm	1. +4.00; +4.25	1. +4.25//−6.25 ☞ −7.75
2. 56mm	2. +8.25;+7.75	2. +6.00 ☞ +6.50 //−6.00
3. 72mm/68mm	3. +3.00; +2.25	3. +10.25//−3.75 ☞ −5.25
		4. +2.00//−10.50D ☞ −11.75

page 118
1. −3.59D
2. +10.10D
3. −6.62D
4. −4.00D
5. a. +1.56
   b. +1.56 // −10.06 x180 ☎ −12.06 x090
   c. +1.25 // −8.12 x180 ☎ −9.62 x090 (In some labs this will be rounded up to −9.75.) The power of a lens with the surfaces found in 5c, if made from a material with index of refraction of 1.530, would be −6.87 −1.50 x090.

page 123
1. 4.0mm;
2.a. BC +8.25D:
   b. true curves +7.75 & −5.25
   c. sag_{front} = 6.5mm; sag_{back} = 4.2mm
   d. ct = 4.3mm

page 126
1. edge 3.8mm, center 5.1mm
2. edge 4.7mm, center 6.3mm

Section VI
page 129
1. −6.22 −0.82 x180
2. +10.02 +0.08 x180
3. +4.67 +0.62 x090

page 134

1.glasses

		D	n	VD	h	t	D_1	SM	%
as is	OD	−14.50	1.586	9mm	.012m	.0015	+1.5	0.853	−14.7
	OS	−10.00	1.586	9	.012	.0015	+1.5	0.894	−10.6

magnification difference of 4.1%

a. for Δt: OD 0.1%
b. for Δvd: OD 1.5%, OS −2%
c. for ΔBC: OD .1%, OS −.1%.

Using all of these changes:

		D	n	VD	h	t	D_1	SM	%
iseikonic	OD	−14.50	1.586	8mm	.011m	.0025	+2.5	0.866	−13.4
glasses	OS	−10.00	1.586	11	.014	.0015	+0.5	0.878	−12.2

magnification difference of 1.2%

In Exercise 1 just moving the bevel of the OS 2mm toward the back of the lens, which will move the lens forward and increase the vd by 2mm, will drop the magnification difference significantly. This may be the most practical solution for this pair of glasses.

2.

		D	VD	h		SM	%
	OD	+1.50	0	.003		1.005	0.5%
	OS	+4.50	0	.003		1.014	1.4%

magnification difference of 0.9%

page 137   −2.25 +0.75 x100 $S_1 = -2.25$, $C_1 = +0.75$

$\qquad$ −8.50 +2.00 x144 $S_2 = -8.50$, $C_2 = +2.00$ $\gamma = 44$, $2\gamma = 88$

$\qquad$ C = +2.16

$\qquad$ S = −10.46

$\qquad$ $2\theta = 67.7$, $\theta = 34$, new axis = 134

$\qquad$ new Rx rounded is −10.50 +2.12 x134 or −8.37 −2.12 x044

page 139-140
1. front reflects 4.0%; back reflects 3.8%; total transmission 92.2%.
2. front reflects 5.1%; back reflects 4.9%; total transmission 90.0%.
3. front reflects 6.2%; back reflects 5.8%; total transmission 88.0%.

page 146-147
1 74.8%
2. center: 83.6%;   edge 62.9%
3. a. windshield .778 b. lens during day .403 c. total during day 31.3%
$\qquad$ d. lens at night .751 e. total at night 58.4%

page 149
1. 33°   2. 21%   3. polariscope or colmascope.

page 151
1. 550nm; yellow or yellow-green.

page 154   back vertex power   front vertex power
1.   +0.06D   +0.06D
2.   +5.41D   +5.10D
3.   +10.95D   +10.03D

Section VII
page 163

1.	a	b	c	d	e
p	100	80	60	40	20
q	67	80	120	inf.	−40
M	−0.67	−1	−2	n/a	2
I	−13	−20	−40	n/a	40

2.	a	b	c
p	80	40	20
q	−27	−20	−13
M	0.34	0.5	0.65
I	7	10	13

3. $1/f = 0 = 1/p + 1/q$; $1/p = -1/q$; $p = -q$; $M = -q/p = (-q)/(-q) = +1$.
4. The image forms to the left of the mirror, it is inverted, real, and magnified.

page 167.

	1.	a	b	c	2.	a	b	c
p		100	40	20		80	60	20
q		67	inf.	−40		−27	−24	−13
M		−0.67	n/a	2		0.34	0.4	0.65
I		−13	n/a	40		`7	8	13

page 175

question 1					question 2			
D_1	+35D	D_F	+36.02D		r_1	+0.02m	D_F	+17.50D
D_2	+1D	f_1	28mm		r_2	+0.05m	f_1	57mm
n	1.50	D_B	+191.91D		n	1.50	D_B	+140D
t	0.035m	f_2	5mm		t	0.05m	f_2	7mm
r_1	+0.014m	D_{eq}	35.18D		D_1	+25D	D_{eq}	23.33D
r_2	−0.5m	f	28mm		D_2	−10D	f	43mm
		OC	1mm				OC	−33mm

page 179-180 (All measurements are in mm.)

lens 1: $D_{eq} = 35.18D$, $f = 28mm$ lens 2: $D_{eq} = −22.84D$, $f = −44mm$

	p	q	M	I	p	q	M	I
a.	60	53	−0.88	−13	60	−25	+0.42	+6
b.	28	infinity	na	na	30	−18	+0.59	+9
c.	15	−32	+2.2	+32				

page 184

n_1	1.00	D_B	+75.56D		
n_2	1.70	f_2V_2	20mm	p	50+13 = 63mm
n_3	1.50	D_F	+40D	q	63mm
t	20mm=.02m	f_1V_1	25mm	IV_2	63+13−18 = 58mm
r_1	0.0175m	D_{eq}	+40D	M	−1.0
r_2	inf.	f_1H_1	25mm	O	20mm
D_1	+40D	f_2H_2	38mm	I	−20mm
D_2	pl	HN	13mm		

The 20mm high image forms real and inverted, 58mm inside the 1.50 plastic.

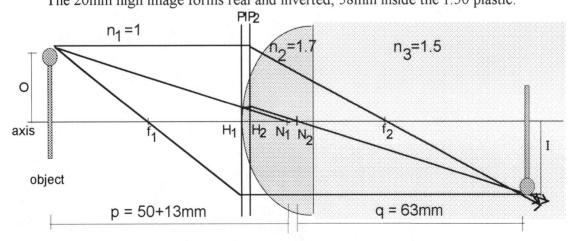

INDEX

sagittal depth (SAG) and, 119-123
Thin lenses and image size and placement, 163-167
    assumptions for, 164
    ray tracing rules for, 165
Thompson's formula for obliquely crossed cylinders, 135-137, 197, 202
Tolerances, 191-195
    base curve, 193
    center thickness, 194
    cylinder axis, 192
    cylinder power, 191-192
    impact resistance, 195
    lens power, 191
    mounted lens, 194-195
    multifocal and progressive addition lens, 192-193
    prismatic power on single lens, 193
    segment position, 194
    UV protection, 194
    warpage and wave, 194
Toric lens surface, 38, 41, 113
    definition of, 190
    flat transposition and, 47
Toric transposition, 115-116
    purpose of, 115
    steps in, 115-116
Toricity of a surface definition, 54
Transmission through absorptive lenses, 142-147
    glass lenses, 143
    Lambert's equation for, 144
    photochromatic lenses, 145-146
    plastic lenses, 142
Transverse wave motion, 9, 190
Trigonometric tables, 203-204
True power formula, 117-118, 202

U

Ultraviolet (UV) protection, requirements for claiming, 194
Ultraviolet speed and wavelength, 12-13, 26

V

V-value, 26
Velocity of waves, 12
Vergence, 13, 14-15
    convergence, 15, 186
    concave lens, 29, 156
convex lens, 28
    definition of, 190
    divergence, 14, 187
    mirrors and changes in, 155-157
    negative, 14, 187
    positive, 15, 186
    reflection from plane mirror and, 155
    refraction through lens and, 28
Vertex distance and effective power, 64-67
Vertex power, back and front. *See* Back and front vertex power
Vertical imbalance, 89-90
    unlike add powers and, 95-97
Vertometer. *See* Focimeter
Vogel's Rule. *See* Base curve

W

Wave formula, 13-14, 202
Wave motion, 9
Wave theory of light, 9
Wavelength, 9
    definition of, 190
    measuring, 11
    computing using diffraction, 150
Waves, properties of, 11-13
    colors and, 12-13
    frequency and, 11
    velocity and, 12

X

X-ray speed and wavelength, 12, 26

Y

Young, Thomas, 150